LIVE
LEARN
LOVE
WELL

LIVE
LEARN
LOVE
WELL

Lessons from a Life of Progress Not Perfection

Emma Lovewell

BALLANTINE BOOKS

NEW YORK

2024 Ballantine Books Trade Paperback Edition

Copyright © 2023 by Emma Lovewell

Published in the United States by Ballantine Books, an imprint of
Random House, a division of Penguin Random House LLC, New York.

BALLANTINE BOOKS & colophon are registered trademarks of
Penguin Random House LLC.

Originally published in hardcover in the United States by
Ballantine Books, an imprint of Random House, a division of
Penguin Random House LLC, in 2023.

ISBN 978-0-593-49737-1
Ebook ISBN 978-0-593-49736-4

Printed in the United States of America on acid-free paper

randomhousebooks.com

9 8 7 6 5 4 3 2 1

Book design by Caroline Cunningham

To my father, Mark Alan Lovewell, and my mother, Teresa Yuan. Thank you for encouraging me to use my creativity, always. I love you.

CONTENTS

LIVE
LEARN
LOVE
WELL

INTRODUCTION

On August 2, 2022, I celebrated my fifth anniversary at Peloton. Though we announced my anniversary ride a week before, we had actually been planning it for months. In one of our scheduling meetings earlier that year, my producer had said, "Your five-year anniversary is coming up, do you want to teach a special ride to celebrate?" Five years. It seemed like both a minute and a lifetime. I thought of how far I'd come in that time, and what everyone had been through in the last few years, all of the hardships and successes I'd heard about from Peloton members, and I thought, *YES.* Never miss a moment to celebrate how far WE'VE come.

As soon as my producer and I started discussing ideas for the ride, I knew I wanted to use the same playlist I'd used during my premiere ride for Peloton, a list I had agonized over five years earlier. Why? Because those songs still have the power to move me; they had been so special to me that I'd picked them for one of the most pivotal days of my life.

As the first strains of "Creep" by TLC came on last August, I felt transported back, not only to 1994 when the song came out but also to that first day in 2017 when my body was vibrating on the platform with nerves, excitement, and anticipation of what was to come. I don't remember much about what I said on my first ride, but I remember *exactly* how I felt. I couldn't believe I was here, in New York, teaching a class I loved to 2,300 people, when the record for live members was 1,000. I had been teaching fitness for a few years but only to 50 people in a room at once.

Peloton was already a thriving company when I joined in 2017. It had been founded in 2012, and I was instructor number eleven at the time. But I was new and I wanted so much from that premiere ride. It was my introduction to this incredibly passionate and engaged group of people, members and employees, and I wanted to show my authentic self. I wanted all of us to finish the ride feeling connected and exhilarated. I hoped that I would be well received. I wanted everyone at home to experience the same brilliant spark of energy and fun that is the power source for my life: to feel free, capable, and resilient, the way I do when I finish a workout. Could I give that feeling to every rider with me that day?

Some of the other instructors were riding in the front row to support me. I remember looking out just beyond my handlebars and seeing Robin, Ally, Cody, Hannah, Jess King, and Christine all beaming while looking back up at me. I was so nervous I could have blacked out, but I knew I was ready for this moment. TLC led into the opening notes of my favorite Janet Jackson song, and they put me right in the groove. A hair flip, then a body roll, and my whole being was moving along to the music. My pedal strokes were right on beat with the bass and I started to fly. I was concentrating so hard on creating a positive experience for everyone that I didn't read even one leaderboard name. To any of you who hit a milestone the day of my first ride, please know I was proud of you . . . even if I hadn't quite mastered how to say so yet! It felt like I was doing a million things at once. I was glancing at my notes to stay on track, tossing out a few words of encouragement, and trying to remember to move my gaze between the camera and the members in the studio.

When that premiere ride was finished, I took a deep breath and wiped the sweat off my face, still buzzing from the thrill of it all. I almost couldn't believe I had had the opportunity to share my passion for fitness with all those people at once. (The number of live riders has gotten much higher in recent years, but at the time 2,300 riders felt like a million.) That initial ride was hard, and I finished it both satisfied with how it had gone and eager to tackle everything I still had to learn. But the very first time I said, "What's up, Peloton, I'm Emma Lovewell!" I felt like I was opening an exciting new chapter in the story of my life, and I couldn't wait to see the rest unfold.

I became a fitness instructor because I believe movement

can change your mood and transform your mindset. My love of movement has been like a thread of positivity running through my life even at my lowest moments. Movement isn't just a must-do for your body; it's like taking a multivitamin for your soul. Don't we all feel like happier (and let's be honest, nicer) people after a workout? *Movement is fun*, especially when you find the kind that's right for you. It's also helped me stay connected to my body, shown me I can do hard things, and encouraged me not to give up when life gets tough.

My story began when two unlikely people met by happenstance on a subway platform in New York City. My music-loving dad, Mark, was waiting for the 6 train after a gig when he encountered my beautiful mother, Teresa, who needed directions. Mom and her family had recently moved to New York from Taiwan to follow the path that they laid out for her. *Study accounting, get a practical job, earn money, marry a Chinese man, and have a family.* Falling in love with my folk-singing, white, Massachusetts-born father wasn't part of that plan. They had to hide their relationship at first. My mother would lie and say she was going to the library when she was really going to see my father. My mom and dad soon moved in together and started building a creative life for themselves. My dad was a musician and writer, and he encouraged and influenced my mother to follow her passion, so she transferred schools and enrolled at Pratt Institute School of Art in Brooklyn to study oil painting. New York City in the 1970s was a fascinating place of contradictions. It was glamorous and gritty, a haven for artists and musicians, a singular time that every dreamer like me probably now romanticizes. I picture them walking arm in arm, Dad with his wavy brown hair and big beard, Mom with her straight black hair that reached the middle of her back. Their own version of John and Yoko, always headed to a Zen meditation workshop or an art gallery or to hear live music. My parents made the most of their time in NYC. My dad would perform at different cafés and bars downtown. To supplement his income he worked at the South Street Seaport Museum as an editorial assistant, and then later at the *New York Post* as a copy boy. He remembers working during the bicentennial celebration at the seaport in 1976, with a parade of sailboats passing by. At the *Post,* he sometimes drove Rupert Murdoch home from the office in the afternoons. My mother, also young and very driven, worked at Time Life in the picture collections department. She would take hundreds of photo negatives and sort them into giant filing cabinets. My parents both worked full-time while attending college full-time. Hustling to make it is in my blood. As aspirational as it sounds to me now, I know it was hard for them too, and, after several years in the big city, they decided to move to Martha's Vineyard. My father's family had been there for generations, and it made sense to raise a family there. Martha's Vineyard can be opulent, but our existence was hand-to-mouth. We were year-rounders, not the wealthy visitors who filled the boutiques and restaurants every summer. Dad was a reporter for the local paper, and Mom took care of my older brother, Alan, and eventually me. She also worked part time in restaurants, cleaned houses, worked as a substitute teacher, and taught the occasional Chinese cooking class in the kitchen of our small house to make ends meet. Money was always tight, and we had to be very self-sufficient. Our family bought clothes and other things we needed at thrift stores. We had a moderate-sized garden where my mother grew vegetables and flowers. Always scrappy, I was taught by my parents that it's important to know how to fix things yourself. Even better? Have the skills to build what you need. Our modest house with its vegetable patch was the opposite of the grand houses on the Vineyard—with their meticulously kept lawns and clear-blue swimming pools. I didn't always know it (especially when other kids had the coolest new toys and jeans that weren't a couple of inches too short), but I had everything I needed. I know the way I talk about the Vineyard makes it seem like a little slice of heaven, and in some ways it is, but so many parts of my life growing up there were challenging, especially in my teenage years when my family came apart (unexpectedly, at least to me) and I faced obstacles and setbacks to my dreams. But I look back on those years and realize that so much of the adversity I faced was forming the core of who I am and giving me the strength to pursue the passions I would eventually discover. I was being handed crucial tools to build a life for myself.

Fast-forward to that Peloton anniversary ride. When you get a moment like that to reflect, you can't help but think about all the twists and turns a life can take; the strange course that brought me from dancing my little heart out on the Vineyard to audition after audition in New York City to years of wandering and wondering where next to take my passions to finally clipping into that bike in front of the whole world! Not to mention all the head-spinning things that have happened in the five years since I joined Peloton. We've been through so much on this bike together: awakenings, celebrations, moments of transcendence, fear, hopefulness . . . we made it through a global pandemic, for goodness' sake! Anniversaries mark the passage of time and *progress* over time, and on this ride the feelings were bigger and better than most I'd experienced in that seat. Same playlist, but this time I was comfortable in my skin and confident in my ability to guide you. I was flooded with pride during that ride, for my teammates and especially for all of you. We've all been on this journey together and have grown together. We have *progressed* together. Progressed. Never perfected. And we keep progressing every time we clip in together.

Do you ever sit back and reflect on your first ride or your early days of discovering movement? What do you remember? Were you a seasoned cyclist ready to jump into action? A newbie nervous about what to expect? No matter where you were in your fitness journey, you were starting a new chapter. You were writing the next part of your story. By incorporating new movement into your life, you were enhancing your own story with promise and possibility.

When I started thinking about writing down my stories, I realized I wanted to share the magic that can happen when movement becomes a major theme in the story of you. In my Peloton classes, I often share tiny anecdotes about myself and about the world from my perspective. It has allowed people all over the globe to feel connected to me virtually. It has surprised me and inspired me. How incredible it is that moments of my life, how I've struggled, overcome, triumphed, and grown, could become a part of other people's stories, that the things I say and do can inspire others to write new chapters for themselves.

My dad always said, "Anyone can be a storyteller." And when I started to think about the things I speak about on the bike, I realized he was right. I am a storyteller, and I'm finally sitting down to write out my experiences at length, instead of five sentences told between breathless interval sets. Like many of you, I've experienced ups and downs. I've woken up in the morning wondering, *What's next?* I know what it feels like to be in flux, untethered, and seeking something that makes the challenges of life easier to face. What always kept me going was my quest to be at peace mentally, emotionally, and physically. And that began with movement, with creating and nurturing a connection between my mind and my body. This doesn't happen overnight, and it's not as simple as checking off items from some healthy to-do list. It's an ongoing process, and I'm here for the ride.

Writing your best life story isn't about punishing workouts and restrictive eating. *Wellness,* to me, is about showing love for yourself through movement, good food, meditation, friendship, love, dancing, laughing, standing up for what you believe in, and being deliberate about what you choose to bring into your life. In this book I'm going to share what I've learned about how wellness impacts your entire story. From gardening lessons and dancing to meditation and traveling, I hope I can show you how that thread of movement has made these stories shine brighter. I'm grateful to be part of your journey. We can celebrate who we are *in this moment* and where we come from (even if that's a difficult story), because it's all part of the amazing person that is *you*. The minute that's happening now is the only one we get! We all have different stories and reasons we picked up this book, but we are united by being here together. Let's acknowledge our accomplishments and see how far our stories can take us.

Live. Learn. Love well.

ONE

Cultivate Gardens for Greater Happiness

Life can move at breakneck speed, and it can be hard to keep up. It often feels like the older I get the faster time goes, and I find myself getting whiplash if I don't remind myself to slow down and just breathe. There are many days where my schedule is packed full and I'm hustling to fit everything in. Did I remember to put my clothes in the dryer? Did I finish my playlist for my upcoming 90s Rock Ride? On my commute to the city there are meetings to schedule, calls to return, and emails to answer before I arrive at the studio for a live ride. I'm sure that most of us are well acquainted with the feeling I'm talking about: It's "overwhelmed" meets "where do I even begin?" This is the challenge that comes along with wanting it all . . . everything can start to overflow, and it can feel like too much. Sometimes slowing down to "smell the roses," combined with a bit of careful pruning, is needed to make it all work smoothly. Every spring, as I start to plan my next garden, I find myself standing in the garden center surrounded by beautiful plants and flowers. I want to buy *everything*. I also know that if I want my garden to thrive, I need to make careful choices about what I decide to plant. Gardens flourish best when they are carefully cultivated, and as I fill my trunk with my final choices, it hits me again that planting a garden is a template for living a well-balanced life. Gardens *and life* benefit from planning, consistency, energy maintenance, and the ability to set limits. Sometimes the most important thing you can do is say, *This isn't working, and it's got to go.*

As you probably know, I could talk about gardening all day every day, but I will spare you the full barrage of my enthusiasm and instead attempt to impart a few crucial lessons from one of my favorite hobbies. Though I had a rocky start with my feelings about gardening, I have come to see that so many of the choices that make a garden thrive are applicable to life writ large, and I often find that things I've learned from tilling the soil go well beyond the garden walls—they help me live with purpose and passion (and can help you too, even if you never pick up a shovel!).

When I'm deliberate about my plant choices and soil maintenance, all the planning, digging, watering, and constant care eventually result in a bounty of fresh vegetables and flowers. It's like I've conjured my own little miracle out of the earth. When my friends and family gather at my table for a late-summer meal, the vases of brightly colored zinnias, the fresh grilled zucchini, the string beans, the jars of cucumbers I've quick-pickled, and the heirloom tomatoes are the result of all my careful decisions. It's not only what I put into my garden that made it flourish, but also *what I took out*.

As I said, my relationship with gardening wasn't always the full-on lovefest you now see on Instagram. For me, gardening was a practical skill that I slowly leaned into loving as an art. When I was a kid, helping my mother with the garden was not only an unpleasant chore but one I was sometimes embarrassed by. I saw the dirt, the constant weeding and watering, the little containers of beer we put out to kill slugs, and the horror that is the smell of homemade compost as pungent reminders that we were different from other families. The worst gardening-related task came every night after dinner, as sure as homework. I'd hear my mother call out to me from the living room.

"Emma! Take this out to the compost."

I'd groan and slowly walk into the kitchen, knowing my mother was going to hand me the unpleasant remainders of my family's dinner. Vegetable ends, scraps of meat (if we ate meat that day), and anything else that was no longer edible were tossed together. Imagine a repulsive salad made from garbage. I'd take a deep breath, grab the unreliable flashlight, open the back door, and walk cautiously across the backyard toward the compost pile. It wasn't just that I found this task gross, I was also worried about what I'd encounter in the ultra-pitch-dark that covers Martha's Vineyard. Skunks and racoons were common, bugs were aplenty, and snakes were a real possibility. I knew monsters weren't real, but this didn't stop me from worrying that some horrifying sea creature had crawled out of the ocean and slithered into my yard and was waiting for a little girl like me to come by so it could swallow me whole. And because my mother didn't mess around, she composted everything (yes, you can compost meat and dairy if you're brave). While this meant less waste and more compost for the garden, it also meant that the smell was next-level awful. As I got closer to the pile, trying not to gag, the smell grew more powerful. Finally, when the odor had reached maximum offensiveness, I'd run toward the pile and fling the nasty contents of my bucket in the general direction of the smell. I'd run back through the yard and breathe a sigh of relief when I was inside, safe from wildlife, monsters, and the almighty smell that is putrid meat rotting amongst many months' worth of vegetable scraps.

Soil without nutrients is useless. Composting is taking old scraps and using them to your benefit. Composting is a great sustainability tool that makes less waste and turns waste into gold. After a successful summer garden my mom would say, "It must be from all the compost we added to the soil!" It was something that I hated but also had to appreciate because it worked. It was valuable trash. Lots of moments in life are similar. Sometimes bad days, gross tasks, or seemingly useless experiences can add up to be really valuable, given enough time. You can't always see, when you're in it, how disparate parts of your life can come together to become useful and meaningful. Sometimes you have to embrace the garbage and hope it becomes something beneficial.

Unlike many people on the Vineyard, our garden wasn't just a luxurious hobby. The hard work we put into our garden wasn't about preserving decades-old hydrangea bushes or tending to the delicate needs of roses that had been planted by someone's great-great-great-grandmother. Our garden was *a necessity*. My parents were committed to eating nutritious foods, and growing our own vegetables made the most sense on a tight budget. Remember, Martha's Vineyard is an island, so whatever you don't grow yourself has to be brought from the mainland to the island grocers. And yeah, that made even the most basic items way more expensive.

Every year my mom carefully plotted out what we would put in each row of her garden—rotating where we put the green beans, tomatoes, and cucumbers to yield maximum results. Not only was gardening a great way to save money, but there were plenty of items my mom would grow that you couldn't even buy at the grocery store. Every spring my mom would order exotic, hard-to-find seeds so she could grow her favorite Chinese water spinach, bok choy, Chinese cucumbers, etc. Each year when the first signs of spring showed up on the Vineyard and Mom dragged me outside to help prep the garden, I couldn't help but think, *Why can't we be like all the other families and just buy everything we need at a real store?* But after months of weeding and watering, lettuce would arrive, zucchini would spring out of their yellow blossoms, bright red peppers and tomatoes would appear, and snow peas would wind themselves around their wooden stakes, dangling off like little prizes. Filling a basket with the foods we had grown ourselves felt magical. We put in the work and now we actually got to eat something our labor and sweat and patience had grown from *nothing.* We had transformed the dirt into the tomato sandwiches and the stir-fried string beans tossed with sesame oil, garlic, and ginger on my dinner plate. As I nibbled on a crisp string bean, salty from the soy sauce, I'd think, *Maybe gardening isn't so bad.* The work was worth it in the end, and maybe it even made the food taste better. Knowing how much effort was put into each vegetable made it even more delicious. (Of course, as a little child I didn't like most vegetables, so that was probably infuriating for my parents! Thank goodness, I learned how to love vegetables as I got older.)

Many years later I was living in Williamsburg, Brooklyn, enthusiastically trying to will my dreams into reality. I had left my college campus for a sparsely furnished third-floor walk-up. It had someone's parents' discarded sofa with a matching chair and a well-loved coffee table that we brought in from the street. In the kitchen there was a slightly wobbly Ikea table with two mismatched chairs, and there was always a small pile of dishes in the sink waiting to be washed. Our basics were covered—my roommate (a friend of a friend) and I had a place to sit and a place to eat. My only contribution to the shared spaces of the apartment was a plant: a hot pink geranium that sat in the windowsill by the kitchen sink, where the sun shone brightest, providing a cheerful spot of green. The plant was a small thing, but it's what made this little apartment in a huge city feel like a home to me. I had left home after graduating from college to pursue a career of some sort—ideally in dance, but I was doing whatever I could just to make ends meet. I was taking small odd (sometimes *very* odd) jobs from Craigslist and bartending at night. When I wasn't working, I was getting to know the city, taking advantage of every opportunity to go out, meet new people, and explore. I recall getting ready in the morning for a full day in the city, printing out directions from Mapquest to every location I needed to be at that day. I'd write down notes and which subway lines I would need to take so I wouldn't get lost. Life before smartphones was definitely adventurous. I kept busy, but the thing about New York City is that you can be completely surrounded by people and still feel lonely or homesick. That single plant gave me a much-needed touch of comfort during my New York City initiation period. The plant served as a happy reminder of where I came from too. After a lifetime of feeling occasionally embarrassed by my parents and their hippie lifestyle of compost and quinoa, I was proud that my family had taken control of our problems and created solutions. As I struggled to find my own path as an adult in a big city, I started to view my scrappy upbringing on Martha's Vineyard as a source of strength. My childhood wasn't something to be embarrassed by—it taught me that I had the power to cultivate any kind of life I wanted.

Over the next few years there were many jobs and several different apartments. In my late twenties, I became friends with a woman named Katie, who worked at the same night-club as I did. We became fast friends at work once we real-ized we had so much in common. Her dad was born and raised in China but moved to the United States, where Katie was raised. She grew up celebrating many of the same holi-days as I did and had many of the same traditions. One of our first times hanging out was when we decided to throw a Lunar New Year party at a hot pot restaurant in Chinatown. Katie is still one of the most important people in my life and is more like a sister to me than anything else. The things we have been through together! We were roommates in New York City for five years, but one of our first homes together was a rent-stabilized apartment in the East Village. Our little apartment was only a half a block away from a real grocery store, which meant no more struggling to carry heavy bags of groceries for several blocks. All New York City apartments have their own quirks, and in this one the bathroom sink was situated directly above the toilet. You could pee and wash your hands at the same time if you wanted to.

But there was something else about this apartment that got me excited. It was a second-floor walk-up, and from out the back window I could see a big, empty concrete courtyard. I wondered if this could be my first New York City home where I had a real garden. I went down to check it out, walking past all the garbage cans and recycling bins. The courtyard was dirty and smelled like garbage, and I wouldn't have been at all surprised to encounter a few rats. But the sun shone brightly down there, and I believed I could transform this space into a garden that fed my appetite *and* my soul. I was determined to make some magic in this neglected little nook of the city. I started watching the pattern of the sunlight out of the back window so I could figure out which plants should go where. I started to visualize what the space would look like transformed. Instead of random pizza boxes and the occasional broken beer bottle, I could see brightly colored pots of peppers and containers of red and yellow tomatoes. I would grow flowers too.

This was also around the same time I met my partner, Dave. We coincidentally first met just a few blocks away from where my parents met in the city. We worked for the same company, and after a friend introduced us, Dave politely asked me if I wanted to go grab a bite to eat. It was ten o'clock in the morning, and I had just taught a fitness class, so I was starving. But let's be honest, even if I wasn't hungry I still would have gone. Dave has a similar love of the outdoors and gardening, so when I had the idea to build this garden out back, he was completely on board to help. This would be the first of many gardens we would build together, each having its own personality, highlights, and flaws, but this first one will be one I always remember. All gardens require hard work, but this one definitely takes the cake.

City gardening comes with its own unique set of challenges, especially when you don't have a car. Lugging home plants from local bodegas and heavy bags of dirt from Home Depot made for an epic journey. I dragged all the supplies out the back door (which I had to prop open with a broken slab of concrete or else I'd be trapped outside) and past the trash cans to the courtyard. I got to work putting seeds in tiny pots so they could grow into seedlings. I cut the tops off recycled five-gallon Poland Spring water jugs and drilled drainage holes in the bottom (hot tip: They are the perfect vessel for growing tomato plants). After a couple of hours kneeling on the hot concrete, potting plants, I encountered possibly the biggest urban gardening challenge: There was no spout for a garden hose (not that I owned a hose). *I have no access to water down here.* Keeping my plants watered would mean multiple trips up and down two flights of stairs carrying heavy buckets of water (this was a true workout), trying not to spill it all over the place. As I left a trail of sloshing water behind me, I started to wonder if I was going to get into trouble. I hadn't asked the super if this was okay. I started to worry my project wasn't feasible. I imagined angry landlords, teams of rats devouring my lettuce, neighbors stealing all my peppers, toxic city rain poisoning it all. I understood how my mom must have felt as she sprinkled eggshells at the base of her plants, determined to deter the slugs who treated her handiwork like an all-you-can-eat buffet. I felt protective of these plants that I was pouring so much energy into conjuring from soil. I was invested in their survival, and it became intertwined with my own. After all, if I could grow a tomato plant in New York City, what couldn't I do?

Every morning I'd pour myself a cup of coffee and look down on my secret garden. Slowly but surely the stalks made their appearances. The tomato plants began to climb and the flowers bloomed, brightening up the drab space. I had multiple flower containers filled with annuals, like marguerite daisies, verbena, multicolored lantana, and bright green potato vines that trailed to the ground. My pepper plants sprouted the most adorable tiny peppers that would soon be fully grown. My herbs thrived from the heat of the concrete— I wouldn't have to buy basil or mint from the bodega all summer long. Recycled glass pickle jars filled with zinnias and sunflowers added a touch of beauty to our otherwise run-down apartment. As August arrived, all the up and down with the heavy buckets of water paid off. I sliced tomatoes, made salads, and stuffed peppers to share with Katie. We had friends over, and I'd make Asian dishes like my mom, proudly proclaiming, "I grew the string beans you are eating!"

Soon September came and the sky started getting darker earlier, but I wasn't quite ready for summer to be over. My garden bounty was shrinking fast. "Dave, I think I picked the last tomato." I held the bright red fruit in my palm like it was a baby chick—adorable, fragile, and something I didn't want to let go of. "Emma, we put so much hard work into this garden and we have eaten amazing food all summer long. It's okay that it's coming to an end. You did it, you made this happen." He understood that this garden meant more to me than flowers and food. I had created my own little oasis. I had proven to myself that I had the power to conjure beauty out of a pot of dirt. I had created something where there was nothing, just like my mom did back home. And in doing that, I'd made it my home.

YOU HAVE THE POWER TO CULTIVATE POSITIVITY IN YOUR OWN LIFE

Spring awakenings come in many forms. We all have that moment when something makes us think, *Wow, spring is finally here,* and it usually has nothing to do with the actual spring equinox. It might be your first al fresco dinner, sleeping with the windows wide open, wearing a lighter coat, or the moment you finally pull those Birkenstocks out of the back of your closet. It's always a positive sign for me when the birds start chirping again, but I think the real sound of spring, to me, is the metal of my shovel breaking through the newly thawed earth. My spring comes the first time I get *really* dirty: dirt on the knees of my jeans, dirt under my fingernails, dirt all over my gardening gloves, and the back of my car is filled up with heavy bags of dirt and mulch. I know it's time for me to plan, reevaluate, and get to work. I kneel in the dirt for hours getting the garden ready, the smell of fresh soil and compost all around me as I pull out rocks and dead leaves. All the digging, shoveling, and watering is hard work, but I know it will be worth it for the bounty it brings me. And even beyond the bounty, it brings me peace. Sticking my hands in the dirt helps me feel grounded, especially when so many things in my life feel "up in the air." Walking around my garden every single day to witness the tiny changes that happened overnight is like a meditation to me. It's so simple, and so effective.

As I turn over the soil, I think carefully about what I want to cultivate in my next garden. *Seeing vases of flowers all around the house was delightful; I definitely want to keep growing flowers. The kale got buggy; how can I prevent that? I'll rotate the peppers, beans, and tomatoes—those are always a hit, and I love having extras to give to friends. The herbs are important too; I use them in everything. The melons were a big fail, so I'm not going to take up room with those next year.* A thriving garden requires careful choices. Deciding where I want to direct my energy is as important as the soil, sun, and water. While I believe this is a good plan for gardening, it is also a blueprint for a well-lived life.

Cultivation (in gardening and in life) can be a slow and sometimes difficult process, but it can also guide you to what you want most in life. We all have those moments when we feel depleted, like we need something to lift us up and restore our energy. These feelings are a sign that we need to look inward and make sure we are directing our energy to the right places. To live fully it's important to think about what you need to cut out, what you want to change, and how you want to grow. As I prepare my garden, I also make a point of *preparing myself*: Where do I want to put my energy, and what do I need to cut out? It's like spring cleaning for the soul, and there are a few ways to approach this.

THE PRACTICE OF DEADHEADING

My mom, now a professional gardener, showed me how with one snip of the clippers you could remove something dead so that a plant could redirect its energy. After a flower has blossomed and then turned brown and wilted, that flower must be eliminated so the plant can redirect its energy into growing a new flower. Deadheading is simply removing the dead flower that has already had its moment in order to allow more flowers to shine. A plant will still grow without deadheading, but it won't have as many flowers, or be as prolific, bright, and beautiful. Almost as soon as my mom taught me this form of plant maintenance, I drew the comparison to my own life. Make a point of observing the areas in your life where something is dragging you down and depleting your energy. Maybe an area in your life once deserved your full attention and energy, but it's already had its moment. Maybe a dream has passed and it no longer serves you; it only drains you. There are many things that could be cut away, allowing you to preserve your energy and give it to something new, making room for another dream to fully blossom. It could be an old relationship or habit that no longer works for you. Hitting the snooze button too many times in the morning, staying in a toxic relationship, or saying yes to people even though you don't have the bandwidth: These things can leave you frazzled or depleted. If you can eliminate them, it allows you to be more productive in your day, put more energy into the positive relationships in your life, and/or spend more quality time with your family.

You deserve to be surrounded by people who make you feel energized, excited, loved, and confident. Do the people you spend your time with create these feelings in you (at least most of the time)? If not, are they the best place to direct your energy? Bottom line: If something is draining your life force, cut it out like a withered rose and watch new growth appear.

THE MYTH OF THE GREEN THUMB

I often hear "I want to have a garden, but I've killed every plant I've ever had. I guess I just don't have a green thumb." Whenever someone says this to me, I can't help but think of all the plants I've killed over the years. There was the lavender plant that withered away two weeks after being planted, and the rhododendrons that lost all of their leaves. I have watched more plants die than I can remember. Most frustrating are the peace lilies I've tried to grow indoors that are generally considered "easy to care for." They start off with shiny green leaves and those beautiful white blooms, and then I swear I watch them wither away in front of my eyes. No matter what I do, I cannot keep a peace lily alive. It's not that I've done something wrong; some plants simply don't make it. It's part of the gardening cycle. Some things thrive when others do not, but let me be clear . . . your thumb has nothing to do with it!

My advice to anyone who wants to start a garden is this: Start off slow. Don't go crazy ordering seeds from catalogs and transforming your entire yard into a vegetable garden. That's a ton of work, and while it is satisfying work, I believe it's best to start small and grow bigger as you learn the ropes. Start with just one plant like I did. Buy a geranium or a basil plant and stick it in your sunniest window. Water it and let it be until the soil dries out and it needs to be watered again. Experience the gratification of watching something grow, whether it's a bright pink flower or some fragrant herbs for a Sunday tomato sauce. Channel that success into a few more plants, a window box, or a container of tomatoes on your back porch or fire escape. Enjoy the process and see where it takes you.

FLOWERS DON'T BLOOM OVERNIGHT

Growing a garden takes time, especially when you're adding big perennials like lilacs, hydrangeas, or rhododendrons.

Rarely do I stick a big plant in the ground and think, *Ta-da! My work here is done!* I know it will likely be several years before my plants really pop. Plants need time and care to adapt to their environment before they reach their full potential. And sometimes we need to accept that certain things happen at their own pace, and we should make a point to appreciate each stage along the way. Some rhododendrons only grow a single foot in ten years, but that doesn't mean their bright purple blooms are any less beautiful. There's a rhododendron in British Columbia that's about 26 feet wide and 30 feet tall that bursts out with about 4,000 blossoms each spring and *it took about 115 years to get to this size.* While this plant must be spectacular to look at, there is no point in comparing it to its smaller counterparts. Each plant is at a different stage in its life, just as we are all at different places in our lives. Where we are today isn't necessarily where we will be a few weeks, months, or years down the road. Whatever your goals are, whether they are about fitness, success, careers, or relationships, it's important to give yourself credit for every step forward. A gradual change is still a change. I'm a big believer in loving yourself to success, and that requires being kind and patient with *yourself.* You cannot hate yourself into change; you must love yourself into greatness. Give yourself the time and care you need to really blossom into the best version of you.

We all need different things to reach new heights. I've learned over the years that being around other creative people is my very own version of sunshine, water, and good soil. I also require regular exercise, vegetables, my partner, Dave, meditation, laughter, cats, my family, dancing, art, visits to the ocean, traveling, music, and my entire Peloton community (you boost my spirits every day). I know how it feels to get stuck, and sometimes I still curl up on the couch to binge reality TV and eat a pint of Ben & Jerry's ice cream. But after years of cultivating my garden *and my life,* I do know the basics of what I really need to thrive. If you feel like something is standing between you and massive growth, it might be time to get dirty. Dig into the raw materials of your life. Make decisions about where you want to foster growth and what needs to be cut away. Be observant, look for places where the sun shines brightest in your life, and seek out what nurtures you. You can have many different gardens, *but you only get one life to tend.* Make it big, make it beautiful, but, most of all, enjoy your time in the dirt.

TWO

Your Voice Is Your Power

When I'm on the bike, guiding you through a ride and urging you to tap into your energy source *because I know you can get up that hill,* you're seeing the assured, confident version of me. My words of encouragement flow naturally and easily during a class, but I didn't always know how to use my voice to inspire people. There were many years when I associated "being quiet"—keeping my thoughts, wants, opinions, and ideas to myself—with "being good." I thought this was how I was supposed to be in the world: passive, small, and even compliant. It took many years and many eye-opening experiences before I discovered that my voice was a source of power within myself and that I could also use it to motivate people to become the best versions of themselves. I didn't always know that what I had to say mattered, and my life changed drastically when I discovered it did. I don't think I'm alone in this struggle, but I want you to know that growth and abundance can happen when you break your silence, speak out, and show the world how valuable your thoughts really are.

There was a time when my partner, Dave, and I left New York City and headed west (making several stops along the way—more on those later). It was a challenging time for me. I was between jobs and not sure what was next. We headed to California, a place we had both been curious about. I liked the idea of being close to my older brother, Alan, who lived there and owned a seafood business, Real Good Fish. I imagined California as possibility in the form of sunshine, palm trees, orange and lemon groves, and an entirely different ocean. There was much to love, but it soon became clear that leaving New York City wasn't a simple solution to all my problems. They came with me. I was working sporadic hours as a personal trainer at a tech company's on-site fitness center, being paid slightly more than minimum wage, and feeling just as adrift as I had before. There were also new challenges in the form of traffic, a long commute, relentless rain, mudslides, and living in an Airbnb where our bedroom *did not have a window*. My career in fitness all of a sudden seemed like the most challenging aspect of my life, and I doubted I had made the right choice. I knew what I wanted from life, but I didn't know how to get it. I took advantage of this time in California to get more fitness certifications and hone my skills. I loved getting to spend so much time with my brother, Alan, and his wife, Jenn, as well as some Vineyard friends who had moved out there as well. We ate well and had incredible family meals together, epic bike rides along the Pacific Coast, and lots of camping trips. It was a time of incredible highs and drastic lows, and even though I had a great partner and positive relationships with friends and family, I still craved work that I felt passionate about. I had clarity about which direction I wanted to go, but I didn't know how to forge ahead. Sitting in our damp, airless apartment (where on earth was all the California sunshine?) eating the free food I was permitted to take from my training job, I felt so low. It was almost like I had allowed myself to be blown backward. I was so exhausted from being adrift, and I longed to just feel like I was on solid ground. I looked at Dave and said, "Why are we here? I miss New York. I feel just as stuck as we were before."

The fitness job at the California tech company was fine, but in reality, I was spending three hours a day in my car commuting there to train only a few people. It dawned on Dave, and eventually me, that there was another tech company, back in New York, ironically, that was really taking off. I had acted in a Peloton Kickstarter campaign video when Peloton was in its very early stages. I hadn't heard of the company when I agreed to the job back in 2012, but I'm so glad I did it. On set, I met the whole team, which was incredibly small at the time, including the CEO, John Foley. I remember John telling me at the shoot, "You're going to love riding on this bike; it's like riding on a cloud!" I left the shoot that day noticing how incredibly kind and driven that whole team was. I remember saying to John, "Best of luck!" I had kept a curious eye on them ever since, watching their success through news articles and TV features. Dave has always been one of my greatest advocates, and he understood how badly I wanted to inspire others to move their bodies, reach their goals, and feel good about themselves. "Emma, why don't you email the CEO of Peloton? Congratulate them on their success; maybe they'll have an opportunity for you." I admit I was a little scared by Dave's suggestion. Just reach out to a CEO? I could think of a million reasons why I shouldn't do this—he'd be busy! He wouldn't remember me! Who am I to ask a CEO if there's a job for me? But also, really, how long could I stay afloat if something didn't change? I wrote an email, just as Dave suggested, congratulating John on all of his success and asking if there were any job opportunities at Peloton for me. I was terrified to click Send. I was flooded with doubt. I hedged. I stalled. But I finally took a breath and sent that email. I was shocked to find a response from John in my inbox twenty minutes later. My career didn't change instantly with one email, and there's a lot more to this story (which we'll get to), but it was that simple act of speaking up and making a case for myself that set things in motion for me. My reluctance to reach out to someone could have cost me the opportunity of a lifetime. Asking for what *I wanted* in that moment was one of the most important things I've done, as it put me on the path to a career that I love and showed me that my voice has value. Many times, we don't speak up because hesitation and fear stops us dead in our tracks—even if what we want is visible just a little way down the road. My quiet years lasted way too long. In fact, the first time I tried to express myself in a big way as a child, I didn't make a single sound.

The Rules of Lip Synching by Emma Age 9

1. Pick a song most people have heard before.
2. No holiday songs. Ever.
3. Do not attempt a duet by yourself!
4. Don't choose an extremely long song; you don't want people to get bored.
5. Use a song that has vocal aerobics or long, drawn-out notes for extra drama.
6. Have all your choreography memorized, so you don't even have to think about it.
7. When planning your choreography, study the way the artist moves and try to mimic their movements. Match your gestures to the lyrics. Practice!
8. Your costume should make you feel confident and comfortable, but also give a nod to the artist.

Long before glittery, gorgeous drag queens regularly "lip synched for their lives" on television, a little girl on Martha's

Vineyard reigned supreme as queen of her own living room. I was shy and reserved, but put a Mariah Carey cassette into the tape player and I'd shed my inhibitions like a dirty sweat-shirt. After hearing the first few bars of "Emotions," the girl who could always be counted on to say please and thank you and do her chores without complaint (most of the time) transformed into a mini pop star. The entire living room was my stage—the coffee table and old wooden rocking chair pushed aside so I could freestyle my moves while doing the classic "my hairbrush is now a microphone" trick. I bopped around the room, my audience consisting of only Mom's large Buddha that was perched on top of the bookcase and my childhood cat, Lucky. I dramatically contorted my face as I pretended to hit F7, Mariah's iconic "whistle register" high note (I'd heard that the only other creature on earth capable of hitting this note was a dolphin).

Head-over-heels in love with Mariah, I was thrilled when my dad offered to take me to Aboveground Records, our town's music store, on my ninth birthday. This trip was spe-cial because I was allowed to pick out anything I wanted as a birthday treat. Dad went off to check out the folk music and jazz sections while I pushed past a group of local kids in flan-nel channeling Kurt Cobain and made a beeline to new re-leases. It's like I was magnetically pulled directly to the Cs, where Mariah Carey's album *Music Box* awaited me like a prize.

I was obsessed with this ultra-successful, feminine (yet not overly girly), mixed-race woman who stood shoulder to shoulder with Celine and Whitney, and Mariah's vocal aerobics and the squiggly sound of a tape rewinding became the soundtrack of my life. Dancing and singing (even faux singing) freed up something inside of me; it was like I was taking a break from being the good girl without actually being bad. I was a solid student, but not a prodigy—there was no advanced calculus or ancient Greek in my grade school career. I was the definition of the kid who does what she's supposed to do, and as a result I flew right under everyone's radar. My guidance counselor noticed though, and she asked me to stop by her office one day. She suspected I might have been having a hard time with some of the other girls and wanted to encourage me to speak up for myself.

"Emma, you're a really good student, but you need to use your voice. You need to learn to speak up if you really want to succeed in life!" She was echoing something I had already heard at home.

My mother may not realize it, but she was born a rebel. The youngest of six children in Taiwan, my mother strayed far from the expectations her family set for her. She moved to New York City in her late teens to go to college. She studied accounting—a practical and solid degree her family readily approved of. What they did *not* approve of was the complete one-eighty that took place once my mother was unleashed into the biggest city in the United States. Not long after meeting my father on a subway platform in Greenwich Village, she transferred to Pratt Institute to study art, got married (to a white man), and moved to an island that was plopped in the ocean four miles off the coast of Massachusetts. This unexpected series of fortunate events was not met with approval by her family. Her actions were viewed as defiance in a culture where women were not encouraged to push against norms. Mom did *exactly* what she wanted to do, even though she hadn't been able to vocalize her desires to her family before she did them. Because of the disconnect my mom experienced between what she wanted and what was wanted *for her*, she pushed me to be my own person—no matter who that was. The island my mom grew up on couldn't have been more different than mine. The cultural expectations my mom faced in Taiwan didn't exist on Martha's Vineyard. But I had a shyness that kept me from using my voice the way my mom (and apparently my guidance counselor) wanted me to.

I left the guidance office and walked down the hallway to chorus, anxiously twisting my mood ring around my finger. How could I have done something wrong just by being quiet? I walked into the chorus room and took my usual seat next to Jessica Olmstadt. As I was rummaging through my backpack, Jessica noticed my mood ring. "Emma! Look. Your mood ring is green. *Oooooooooh.* That means you are JEALOUS!! Who are you jealous of, Emma?" Jessica giggled, and other kids in the class turned to look at my hand as if it had sprouted tentacles. Now the entire chorus was laughing along with Jessica, probably thinking I was jealous of her, because everyone knew she had tons of video games at her house. I looked at my hand; and the stone wasn't even green. *You need to learn to speak up.* "Actually, it's not green, Jessica! *It's blue!*"

Suddenly I became aware of two things: (1) I was standing, and (2) everyone, including our teacher who had just walked in, was staring at me. "Is something wrong, Emma? Why are you shouting? Please take your seat and be quiet." I sat down, 100 percent positive that the color of my face was *red*. If this is what happens when you speak up it didn't seem worth it, and I never wanted to do it again. I had drawn so much attention to myself, and I wanted to disappear under my chair. I struggled to pay attention for the rest of the class, until Mr. Wilson made an announcement at the end: "Reminder, people! The annual lip-synching competition is coming up next month! As third graders you are now eligible to participate." Now this was something I could do, and I wouldn't have to say a thing.

I had always liked the lip synch contest, and I had seen my older brother compete in it with his friends several times. They did a performance one year to They Might Be Giants. They'd take over the stage, all of them dressed in flannel shirts and faded jeans (grunge rock fashion was at its peak), their floppy hair flying as they pretended to jam on invisible electric guitars. I watched these shows with such an intense level of attention you'd think I was a judge on my very own nonexistent reality show. I made mental notes about what I thought worked and what didn't. Just standing there while you lip synched a ballad was so boring. Performing both parts of a duet was amateur hour as far as I was concerned—it never worked. But the worst mistake was when contestants thought they could improvise dance moves. I vowed to myself that I'd never just "wing it" when it came to choreography. I took dance lessons, I knew better. If I planned my choreography and practiced, my dancing could be the thing that set me apart from everyone else. My dance moves could be my ticket to gold.

As I stood backstage the day of the competition, I was nervous—I had never performed in front of this many people before. My dance and piano recitals were much smaller. I had also decided I wouldn't wear my new glasses for my performance. A few months before, I had thought I would look cool in glasses, and I told my parents they needed to take me to the eye doctor because I had *accidentally looked directly into the sun*. But I hadn't needed to make up a silly excuse, because it turned out my vision was terrible. The eye doctor walked me over to the window of her office. "Emma, pick a spot in the parking lot and keep looking at it." I focused on a distant red blob. When the doctor placed the glasses on my face the blob miraculously transformed into a car. All this time I had been throwing dodgeballs randomly, not hitting anyone *because I didn't know that I couldn't see?* On the day my parents took me to pick up my pink and purple floral-print glasses, I was bouncing around with excitement. My glasses were a thing of beauty, and I felt like wearing them would be like getting an instant makeover. But in my heart I knew I could not channel Mariah in my beloved new glasses. There was nothing about them that suggested *hot-90s-pop-star-goddess,* so they had to go. I'd be performing in front of the entire school blindly but exhibiting a more Mariah-like vibe.

I took my position center stage, and as the lights hit me and the song opened with some soft vocalization I felt as comfortable as I did in my parents' living room. I was *in charge.* I felt powerful in my turquoise bodysuit, black vest, and black jeans. The song transitioned to an upbeat tempo, and I launched into my dance routine, executing turns and flipping my newly blow-dried extra fluffy hair. I mouthed the words, even though the lyrics about having a boyfriend were like a foreign language. I dazzled the audience with dance moves inspired by Paula Abdul and Janet Jackson. I made a point to *really connect* with the audience, attempting to make eye contact, even though I couldn't really see. I did spins across the stage, landing in a diva-like pose—hand on one hip, waving a finger as if the audience had done something naughty, expertly mimicking Mariah's signature vocal aerobics, then stuck my arm up in the air in a victory pose to cheers and applause. If I had known about mic drops, I would have dropped mine. I wiped the sweat from my brow and exited the stage where my pink and purple glasses were waiting for me. I put them back on. I was myself again, but this time I was a first-place lip-synching champion, and I didn't have to make a sound.

While I had proven to myself that I could make an impact *without using my voice at all,* my father, a reporter for the local paper, *depended* on his voice to make an impact. I was often Dad's sidekick when he was working on a story, and I was so quiet people barely registered that I was there. I'd stand next to him holding the tape recorder while he effortlessly jumped into a conversation, drawing out a story and collecting facts. I was always amazed at how my dad transformed these conversations into stories that would land on the front page of the *Vineyard Gazette.* And it was while we were out "on assignment" to find a princess that I finally got to meet my favorite pop goddess.

Summer 1994, the island was abuzz—President Clinton was visiting, and rumor had it that Princess Diana was on the island too. Dad invited me to go out on assignment with him, and as we were passing the Oyster Bar, a woman ran out and said, "Mariah Carey is eating dinner in there!" I couldn't have been more excited if Santa Claus himself had appeared and told me Christmas was every Saturday and nothing was off the wish list, not even ponies or backyard swimming pools. My pop icon was a few feet away! I looked at my dad, who simply handed over his reporter's notebook and a red felt pen. Dad gently pushed me toward the door of the restaurant. "Go meet her!"

As a tiny kid, walking alone through the door of that loud

and crowded restaurant terrified me, but I stayed focused on my mission. As I made my way toward the back of the restaurant, it was like the crowd parted just for me . . . sitting there with her then-husband at a table for two, in a navy and white sailor dress, hair flowing down her back like a breezy river, was MARIAH HERSELF. She practically glowed. I approached her table and stood there with my notebook and pen, saying nothing—I couldn't get my voice to work. Mariah smiled at me. "Are you our waitress for tonight?" I smiled back and hopefully handed over the pen and paper. Mariah kindly signed her name for me, a little girl who never said a single word to her. The stars might have aligned for me that night at the Oyster Bar, but silent staring can't reliably be counted on if you really want to make your mark.

That little girl who always said please and thank you grew into a hardworking, dependable woman who never made a fuss. Even in adulthood, I continued to associate being quiet and being grateful with *being good*. "That doesn't work for me" or "I'd prefer this" were phrases that just didn't come out of my mouth. When I was bartending in New York City right out of college, I didn't say a word when I was scheduled for the shitty, low-tip shifts even though I had seniority. Doing my job meant sucking it up. We all have breaking points though, and mine came at an after party during New York City's Fashion Week. A friend and I were chatting with a seemingly high-profile woman who mentioned she regularly traveled to China for work. Between sips of champagne and quick stories about the sights she'd seen, she looked right at me and said, "The thing about Chinese people is that they are so two-faced . . . they'll stab you right in the back." My face went blank. *Did she just say that?* Before the racist remark could fully register, my friend said, "Emma is Chinese." A cloud of embarrassment washed over the woman's face as she made an excuse about seeing a friend across the room and scurried off. I spent the rest of the party in a daze, like I had been sucker punched. What she said hurt, and knowing that I didn't respond to this racist comment was like dumping a pile of salt in a wide-open wound.

On my way home that night I was full of regret. I didn't stand up for myself, and I didn't stand up for my mother, my brother, and the rest of my family (not to mention the literal billion other Chinese people in the world) by calling this woman out for her racism. I should have said something. I thought back to that little girl who was so comfortable with her silence that she became the most decorated lip-synching champion of her school (I won every year from third through eighth grade, except for the year my parents got divorced and I did not participate). That girl had wanted to express herself, but movement was the only way she knew how to do it. Didn't I owe her something now? Would my third-grade self have looked at me in that moment and thought, *Are you seriously going to let that fly? You come face-to-face with a racist comment and you don't take action?* It was time for me to start making some noise. That was the day I vowed to see where my voice could take me.

WORDS ARE POWERFUL

The email to Peloton that I was afraid to send eventually landed me here, where I have used my voice to connect with people from all over the world. When I sit down at my kitchen table to create a playlist and plan my rides and strength classes, it's you I have in mind. I want everything I say to matter. My choices are intentional. I think about experiences that have altered me, and I try to transform those moments into stories that inspire and teach. I pick words that will encourage and provide a bit of solace to get through the tough spots. I want to make people feel good about their time with me and be proud that they showed up for themselves.

But what I didn't expect was how much your voices would mean to me, how much your words would fill my heart with gratitude and inspiration. A father wrote to me to share that he recruited a group of his friends to ride with him in support of his daughter's cancer treatment. A nurse who recently lost her mother got in touch with me to tell me how much my rides have helped her through her grief. These stories serve as a perfect reminder of why I have devoted my life to wellness and fitness. Words can be the spark that ignites someone's inspiration . . . it can be something as simple as giving a high five to a rider hitting a milestone or encouraging a friend to show up for class. We all have our dark days, and the smallest bit of encouragement can be as comforting as a warm blanket. A single word from you has the power to alter someone's day or impact their next step. Every day brings another opportunity to make someone feel good and smile. While I like to take advantage of these little moments to spread joy and be a positive force, there are other important ways to utilize your voice.

CREATE THE CHANGE YOU WANT

I found my voice gradually. I didn't wake up the morning after that party where I heard the racist comment able to change the world, but after seeing how much pain a few words could inflict, I understood how much impact a single voice can have. Over the last few years, I, like so many others, have been horrified by the violence being perpetrated against people of Asian descent, especially in New York City, where I had always felt welcome and safe. Only a few blocks away from where I work, an elderly Asian woman was attacked, and I experienced a fear I hadn't known before. I knew I had to speak out when I realized I was afraid to let my mom, who was visiting, walk the few blocks between the Peloton studio and Hudson Yards. Though it's something so many people of color experience daily in this country, it was the first time I felt that my mother and me and every other person of Asian descent were not safe.

I spoke out in rides and on social media, using whatever kind of platform I had access to in order to raise awareness about the rise in this kind of bias crime. After celebrating my Taiwanese heritage on my Lunar New Year ride, I received an outpouring of support and gratitude from the Asian American community. I was amazed when my words on this ride led to a huge opportunity for me to go to Capitol Hill (virtually) to talk about the violence and racism directed toward Asian Americans. Once-quiet-me was going to Zoom into the offices of the U.S. Congress to speak with elected officials and lobby in support of a bill to protect people against COVID-19 hate crimes, called the COVID-19 Hate Crimes Act. I was informed by Peloton's Government Affairs staffer that I could have ONE MINUTE to express my feelings and thoughts, so I had to prepare to speak up loudly and clearly. Racist violence, of any kind, is totally unacceptable. I was told how to properly address senators and members of Congress and to speak from the heart. When it was my turn, I talked about how my mother emigrated to New York City when she was eighteen years old and how she started her own business in her fifties. I shared how I see my mother as the embodiment of the American dream, and that she's been a huge source of inspiration for me and my brother. I explained that I was proud of how Peloton, which has two Asian cofounders and many employees and members, was raising awareness of this issue and donating money. I wrapped up by respectfully urging that Bill S937, the COVID-19 Hate Crimes Act, be passed immediately. I was thrilled when this bill did pass, and I'm proud that my voice was part of the process. Its passage was a small victory, and there is so much work to be done to protect so many other marginalized communities facing bias crimes and racist violence, but I was honored to be able to use my voice as a catalyst to change at least one thing that I knew wasn't right. It is easy to think that we are a lone voice in a sea of many and that we'll never be heard. I have felt that way. But when you care deeply about an issue, speaking up is the only chance you have at contributing. When you speak up for yourself or others, whether it's responding to a quick and sharp racist comment or a lifelong quest to create change, voicing your thoughts is the first step toward finding a solution. No action can be taken if you remain silent. You can't know what effect your words will have, but there is always an impact, big or small.

OWN YOUR WINS

During my five-year-anniversary ride, I took a moment to reflect on some of my proudest moments at Peloton. I am proud every time someone crushes their core (or crushes their core two). I'm proud of creating the listening parties where I share my love of new artists, developing the artist series rides, and launching Dance Cardio and Pilates. The success of these endeavors has taught me to trust myself fully, that my ideas have value. There's a tendency when cataloging your accomplishments to worry that you're bragging, but if you don't shout out about your wins, who will? Not every venture will result in brag-worthy successes, but your wins are yours to own. Be loud when it comes to your achievements. It can feel scary, but as you toss your wins out into the world, you're announcing, *This is what's important to me, and this is what I've accomplished.* Shout about your wins both big and small, because your value deserves to be seen and celebrated.

Sometimes I think back to the lip-synch rules I wrote when I was nine. I had carefully planned what I'd need to do to win that contest, but I hadn't given a single thought to the value of my own voice. I might have been silent, but there was noise inside of me that wanted to be let loose. And while finding my voice has been life altering, I still think about that quiet little girl standing center stage. She was in her element, but only for a short while. I want to say to her, *How do you feel right now? Free, open, confident, and in control? This is the real you! You don't have to be center stage with a light shining on you to be seen and respected. You can walk off this stage and speak your mind. You can share your ideas, thoughts, frustrations, and dreams, because what you have to say matters. You might be a lip-synching champion, but your silence can only take you so far. If you want to succeed, let go of the silence, shed the self-doubt, and don't hold back. Tell the world loudly and clearly that from now on you're going to be the real you.*

THREE

Make the Conditions Work for You

The first time I came in to work in Manhattan after the pandemic had shut everything down, I couldn't believe it was the same city. I navigated my car toward Hudson Yards, where the new Peloton studios are located, shocked by how quickly things had changed. Driving in New York City is usually a practice in patience, but that day it was fast and easy because there were no other cars. The shops and cafés that were always bustling with energy were abandoned. Many of the storefronts were boarded up as if bracing for a storm. I arrived at the new Peloton studio, where I had never filmed a live class before. It had been scheduled to open the same week that it had to be closed. I was about to do my first live studio ride since the shutdown, and I was shooting it in a place totally new, and totally, eerily, empty. I walked into our new dressing room, a place that had been designed to feel like home, and I fiercely missed my teammates. Our old building on Twenty-third Street was always full of life. All the instructors shared a single, tiny dressing room where we'd laugh and talk while doing our hair and makeup. It was a fun, comforting, and safe space for us. Alone in this unfamiliar setting, I would have even welcomed the smell of our collective dirty laundry.

During the shutdown, the only way to safely get live studio classes up and running was to divide the instructors and their producers into "pods" to minimize contact and exposure. I'd been instructed not to touch anyone (I'd set up my own mic), keep six feet away, and leave my mask on until I started my ride. Live rides before the pandemic were filled with riders and always vibrating with energy, and although I was used to filming alone during our coach-to-camera classes, this was different. I felt truly "alone" (I was so grateful for the few crew members present, who did their jobs so brilliantly). Even more unsettling, now that I was back at work I had chosen to stay by myself at a friend's empty house in Connecticut. Dave and I had been staying at his mother's house, and I didn't want to put them at risk in case I was exposed to the virus. I felt isolated and lonely. As I secured my mic, I caught a glimpse of the instructor's bike, spotlighted alone in the center of the studio. I could never have imagined that this was how my first ride in this state-of-the-art space would go. Instead of being excited, I was afraid and anxious. I walked out to the bike and took a deep breath. I needed to focus before that camera went on. I knew as scared as I was, the people at home, waiting on their bikes for this ride to start, were just as scared, and that many were facing challenges I couldn't even fathom. I wanted to give them support and encouragement during this dark time. The camera went on and I smiled. I tried to leave my immediate world behind so I could connect with you wherever you were. I didn't want to ignore what was happening all around us—but I wanted to be a source of strength for you. The unexpected had happened, and we had all been exhausted by a situation we had no control over. What came to me in that moment was advice I'd heard as a kid learning to sail in the ocean off the Vineyard. *Lean into the wind.* Adjust to the circumstances and do your best to turn them to your advantage. I had some practice with the unpredictable. Sometimes harnessing the wind, and sometimes surrendering to it, can make you stronger and more capable when life throws change your way.

When you grow up surrounded by the ocean, going to the beach is a big part of your life. Mom would get up early on summer mornings and pack enough snacks to last the day— grapes, bright pink cubes of watermelon, peanut butter and jelly sandwiches, and chips. She'd have my brother and me out of the house and on the beach by eight A.M. so we could spend the entire day happily romping around in the sand and surf with other kids. One summer, my mom decided that I should learn to swim, and she signed me up for the free public swimming lessons. I stood on the beach in my little blue bathing suit, freshly covered head-to-toe in sunscreen. The sand was so hot from the midday sun that I had to keep shifting my weight back and forth from my left foot to my right foot. And because it was early in the season, I knew the water would be so cold that standing on the burning hot sand would soon be a relief.

A tall woman in a red Speedo swimsuit approached the group. It was as if Malibu Barbie herself had materialized right there in front of us with a whistle and clipboard. "Hi, everyone! I'm Samantha!" Her smile was enormous, her hair ultra-blond, swept into a bouncy ponytail. Her enthusiasm was practically bubbling out of her—she felt more like a cheerleader than a swimming instructor. "Who here is ready to learn how to swim?" Some of the kids jumped up and down with excitement while other kids clung to their parents, terrified. Malibu Barbie lined us all up near the water's edge and urged us to wade into the surf. A handful of kids ploughed right in, showing no signs of discomfort from the arctic water, while everyone else started shivering the second their big toes got wet. I had no interest in freezing. I stood back. Samantha smiled wildly as she effortlessly bobbed up and down in the waves. "C'mon, Emma, join us!" That's when I did something I wouldn't normally do. I refused. I sat my butt down on the hot sand and watched my fellow classmates.

As the minutes passed by and Malibu Barbie demonstrated

different techniques to stay alive in the massive ocean, I started to feel anxious. I didn't know what to expect next. *What's going to happen? Will I be kicked out of swimming lessons?* As I sat and fretted, the sand started to itch my thighs, and I watched with regret as the rest of the kids (including the ones who had been reluctant to get in) happily romped around in the water. I sat alone and ignored while the other kids seemed to be having tons of fun. I started to wish I had just taken the plunge. So what if the water was cold?

When it was time for the next lesson, fear of being left out overpowered my fear of freezing to death. I marched into that water, Samantha nodding her approval. The water was shockingly cold, but in a few minutes my teeth stopped chattering and I felt *okay* (or maybe my entire body was numb). I followed along with the rest of the class. I kicked and moved my arms just like Samantha, I blew bubbles, and I played games with the other kids. The lesson flew by and none of my fingers or toes had turned blue. As I was toweling off, Samantha walked over to me. She was so tall and pretty; she was like Venus rising from the sea. "Emma! You did a great job today." I swear the warmth of her smile was thawing out my limbs. "I'm so glad you got over your fear and joined us in the water." I looked up at her. "I wasn't afraid. The water was too cold, and I didn't want to get in." She seemed to consider this thoughtfully. "Yes, it can be very cold this time of the year! Sometimes I have to ignore the temperature and just go for it. I think it's great that you didn't let the cold water stop you from having a good time today. You can't learn to swim if you can't get yourself in the water."

Every lesson after that, I'd still hesitate a second or two before I got in the water. Some days I'd be tempted to place my butt back on that warm sand, but I knew in my heart that I wouldn't be able to stand not being capable of holding my own in the ocean. If I wanted to be a strong swimmer I needed to concentrate on the lesson, not the temperature of the water. It was always cold, and I always got over it. I became a very good swimmer who could navigate the ever-changing waters around Martha's Vineyard with ease. I followed in my brother's flip-flops and became a lifeguard, and I also learned to sail. While swimming lessons were a free public offering, sailing lessons were not. The Vineyard Haven Yacht Club offered a junior membership for kids, and my parents managed to find the money for this via a combination of hard work, thriftiness, and a no-nonsense jar my dad placed on his desk at work with a sign that read: HELP EMMA PAY FOR SAILING LESSONS.

Sailing camp started the same way every day. We'd gather in front of the whiteboard to learn about the wind, terms for different parts of the boat, how to tie knots, boat and sail maintenance, and even racing techniques. A few weeks later, I had a killer life-jacket tan and was signed up to participate in my first regatta. My mom had noticed how badly the salt and the lines had cut up my hands, and she got me a pair of sailing gloves. When I slipped those thick, padded gloves onto my small hands before the race, I felt like a real sailor. I was partnered up with my friend Charlee for the race. We took off into the harbor, sailing along smoothly. But when we got into open water we stopped moving. There was no wind. We were dead in the water. Paddling wasn't allowed, so we just sat there. Stuck.

Charlee and I stared at each other. "Emma, the wind has to start up eventually, right?" I nodded hopefully, but it felt like we had been stranded in the sea for hours (it was probably only twenty minutes). I closed my eyes, willing the wind to just blow again. The air responded to my request by remaining as still as a sleeping baby. After another eternity passed by, I noticed Charlee was starting to squirm around. "Emma. Oh my God. I have to pee really bad!"

There are certainly worse places to find yourself without a bathroom, but peeing was nevertheless going to be a challenge. Charlee navigated herself to the stern of the boat and wiggled her butt over the side. I tried not to laugh while Charlee peed, knowing that the roles would soon be reversed if the wind didn't come back. If being stuck weren't enough, another boat from the regatta sailed right past us, laughing and pointing at Charlee while she struggled to get back on board. "Charlee, if those guys got their boat moving, we can too. Let's figure out how to make this work." I frantically tried to remember everything I had learned in sailing camp. Random sailing terms flew through my head, and then I thought about something my teacher had said. "Always remember, you can't control the conditions, but you can make the conditions work for you. There are always obstacles— waves, wind, lack of wind, other boats, and bad weather. A sailor's job is to move forward regardless of difficult conditions." We positioned ourselves to be ready when the wind picked up even the slightest bit, and we were able to make some progress. Then we got stuck again. This pattern of progress-stuck-progress-stuck repeated until we finally saw the finish line. We came in second to last. We were thrilled. We didn't let our panic rule, we took control of the conditions, and we navigated back to dry land. It felt like a big win.

THE CONDITIONS OF LIFE ARE ALWAYS UNPREDICTABLE

There are a million and one things that can keep us from reaching our goals. Think about all the excuses that you create to derail your progress! Maybe you got home late after a nightmare commute and you're tired. There's that mountain of laundry that isn't going to wash itself, and the cookies that need to be baked for the school fundraiser. There will always be something. The conditions of your life are never going to be perfectly aligned with your goals. You must learn to work with the conditions you're in or risk staying put indefinitely. If you want to sail, you don't need to wait for clear blue skies. If you want to improve your wellness and fitness, you can't wait for the perfect time. The conditions do not need to be optimal for you to get stronger. I am not an expert sailor, but crossing the finish line of that race showed me that you *can* take any conditions and make them work for you. It might have taken us hours to finish that regatta, but every time the wind blew, we moved forward. It was far from perfect, but it was progress and that's all you need.

When You're Blown Off Course, Harness the Wind and Look for a New Path

When Dave and I were living in California it was clear we had been blown way off course. We had left our families, our friends, and our apartment behind, thinking we were sailing into smoother waters. But the opportunities and quality of life we'd hoped for just weren't there. It was like I was stuck in that little boat again with no idea how to get back in motion. It was the encouraging response to the email I was afraid to send that gave me the first hint of a light breeze. The CEO of Peloton was glad to hear from me and wanted to connect. That breeze got a little stronger when John referred me to the head instructor and VP of Fitness, Robin Arzon. We got on the phone, and she was happy to talk about her experience at Peloton. Then she quickly added, "By the way, we're not hiring right now." Breeze gone. Stuck again. But as we were wrapping up our call she said, "Send me an audition tape anyway, or next time you're in town come in and audition." I could feel the wind picking up. The offer to audition was a gust I could use to navigate myself to a better place. After auditioning for countless dance jobs, I knew that a video wasn't going to seal the deal. I wanted to grab on to this opportunity, so I booked a trip to New York City.

I immediately met with my longtime friend and fellow cycling instructor Ally Love. I had a plan to dazzle. "Ally, this is what I'm going to do for the audition. I think I'll start right off with a song from Wiz Khalifa and a jog. It will really get things moving." The look on Ally's face gave me pause. "Emma, you're so excited, I can see. But out of the saddle and riding hard on the first song? How about a flat road warm-up first?" I followed Ally's advice and adjusted my sails. I perfected my playlist, choosing a mix of artists that would show my versatility. In addition to the Wiz Khalifa, I had Phantogram and the Foo Fighters. My audition was only fifteen minutes. I wanted to show my range in music taste, along with my personality. With my audition material set, all that was left to do was find the most eye-catching leggings around.

The day of the audition I felt confident; my nerves under control. Before I got on the bike to audition, I took a second to acknowledge the course I'd already charted. The past few months I had been either floating aimlessly or completely stuck, but I had managed to create enough momentum to reach this opportunity. When I finished the audition, I knew in my soul that I had nailed it. That audition was followed by a second interview that was really an entire day of interviews with everyone from producers and the chief content officer to the president of Peloton. While I knew it was going to be an intense day, what I didn't expect was to encounter Cody Rigsby, whom I had known for many years from the dance world. Cody was so thrilled to see me interviewing. He grabbed my hand and dragged me around to every person's desk excitedly, saying, "This is Emma! She's the best. We should hire her!" I was glowing from Cody's warmth and friendship, and I believe the energy he gave me helped get me through that long but exciting day. I wish everyone could have their own personal hype-man like Cody.

After the second interview there were negotiations, contracts, and months of training before I would do my first ride as a full-fledged member of the Peloton family. There was a finish line at the end of my story, and it led me to a big win. I am forever grateful to Ally and Cody for advocating for me, cheering me on, and being in my corner during this time in my life.

Change is inevitable; growth is optional. Opportunities arise at inconvenient times, and difficult circumstances can stall progress. When change hits you in the face, you can try to fight it. But why waste all your energy on a battle you can't win? Use this moment of change as a moment of growth. Can you learn from it? The lesson is the silver lining. Take a breath and see if you can push yourself forward just a bit. Go for a walk, jump on a bike, try a yoga class, and get the momentum going again. It is harder to start moving from a complete standstill than it is when you're already moving.

Keep taking steps forward no matter how small they might be. Soon enough those little steps will lead you to a new course. It might be stall-progress-stall at first, but if you keep working it's going to get smoother. You deserve to see where all that progress can ultimately take you.

Surrender, but Just for a Moment

I follow the same ritual before every live ride. I add electrolytes to my bottle of water, bobby-pin my mic to my head, and put on a quick swipe of lipstick. The last thing I do before I go live is the most important step. I always pause to breathe and feel grateful for the long crazy journey that landed me on the bike, riding with you. This small ritual is a gift to me. It's like surrendering to a gentle wave, taking a moment to breathe it all in and enjoy the place where the current has led me. Working hard to keep your head above water can be exhausting. Creating a ritual to support your voyage can be a huge benefit. Morning rituals are especially important. It can help your day unfold calmly, setting you up for productivity. There are a million ways to embrace a new day. It's important you learn what your own needs are, but there are some components to my morning ritual that serve as mini lifeboats.

Don't Touch That Phone

I'm going to start by telling you what I *don't* do. I do not touch my phone first thing in the morning. Okay, yes, it is my alarm, but after I turn it off, I lie back down with my eyes open looking at the ceiling. I don't need to flood my brain with messages and texts first thing. I do not want to be confronted by demands, obligations, and to-do lists until I'm ready. It's hard; I know that phone is just sitting there waiting to hijack your attention with social media, email, texts, etc., but don't let it! YOU should be your number-one priority first thing in the morning. I give myself at least three minutes to be with myself before connecting with technology.

Hydrate Your Body

Water does a surprisingly good job of helping you wake up, and it's what I reach for right after I get out of bed. Water increases circulation and flushes out whatever was lying around stagnant in your body. Also, you get to give yourself a pat on the back for not starting out your day thirsty.

A Quick Cup of Gratitude

I like to grab my journal, sit down, and just jot down three things I am grateful for (before I get into my to-do list). There's no need to write a novella; this is just for you. Expressing gratitude can give you the strength and confidence needed to manage some tough waters. Gratitude helps keep life in perspective, and acknowledging your privileges helps keep the positivity flowing. It is okay to start with the basics. Writing down *I'm grateful that I'm alive, I'm grateful for this cup of coffee, I'm grateful it's warm outside today*—these are enough to get the positivity flowing. Remember, progress not perfection.

Define Your Goal

I set a single goal every morning. It might be something tangible, like *Today I deal with the ever-growing mountain of laundry that is threatening to take over my entire house.* Or sometimes it's mental, like be extra kind to yourself today. Setting a daily goal isn't necessarily about doing something big like pushing yourself to the next shore. This is an exercise to keep you motivated as you work your way toward that shore.

Stretch and Move

Stretching has been shown to promote healthy blood and lymphatic circulation, two components to a healthy body and mind. Whether you start your day with a yoga practice, strength work, a cycling class, or cardio, movement promotes a clear mind. It helps shed the stress. While a full-length exercise class or workout is ideal, the objective is for you to move in the morning. On a day when I'm not teaching class, I like to do a few stretches and then get into ten to twenty minutes of strength work.

Meditation

Sitting down to breathe through your emotions prevents you from starting your day with a powder keg of bottled-up feelings. Emotions that aren't processed are likely to reveal themselves as you go about your daily tasks. Meditating (even for a few minutes) can be like gliding into a pocket of wind. It can be the element that pushes you forward just when you think you can't move another inch. I will admit that this step is the first thing that gets tossed aside when I'm busy. But I know if I'm feeling off and trying to get back to myself, this step is crucial.

Change can be fun or scary, but it's going to happen whether you want it to or not. So, you have the choice. Do you want to just get blown all over the place, or do you want to harness the wind so you can find your power and move forward? There will be times when you might feel out of control or like you're being held down by a heavy anchor, but those feelings are temporary. What is important is that you try. You show up. You get your butt off the sand and get into the water. There will be obstacles, like cold water or no wind, but you have the chance to either succumb to the challenges or use them as your opportunity for growth. Can you find the little lessons in the challenges? In the end, it's a mindset and it's your choice.

FOUR

Unconditional Love Doesn't Mean Perfection

When I visit Martha's Vineyard, I look up at the night sky and I am flooded with memories. My dad has many interests and talents, including astronomy. When I was growing up, he had a huge telescope, and sometimes he'd wake me up at two A.M. to go outside and watch a meteor shower. Because of my dad, I can identify a handful of constellations, stars, and planets. When I was walking home from town at night as a teenager, after working as a hostess, I'd follow the Big Dipper. It felt like it was keeping me company along the way. When I'm feeling overwhelmed, sad, or uncomfortable, I still look up at the stars. Their presence is a reminder that some things remain constant no matter what you might be facing in life. Change is inevitable, but it's not always welcome. It took one of the most painful times in my life to show me that forgiveness and letting go of the idea of perfection were the keys to finding peace and stability.

When I was twelve years old I came home from school one day and immediately sensed that something was wrong. The energy of the house had changed, and then I found my mom crying hysterically. She told me she needed to go to Dianne's house, and she'd be back in a bit. Dianne is a cousin of my father's to whom my mom had become especially close; she's also my godmother, and incredibly caring and wise. I didn't know what was going on and I was scared. I had sensed tension around my parents, and I'd optimistically thought they were going to tell my brother and me that they were having another baby and were worried we'd be upset. Now it was clear that something else was happening. I started walking around the house, noting that my father's things were missing. Where was Dad's guitar? It was always in the living room. The stack of books he was reading was gone too. I walked into my parents' room and opened the closet; it was half-empty; only my mother's things were left. Next, I opened the medicine cabinet; his things were gone from there too. I was numb as I walked around the house not knowing what to do next.

Thankfully, my brother, Alan, was home. He sat me down on his bed. He said, "Emma, I need to tell you something . . . Dad left. Mom and Dad are getting a divorce."

He walked me to my bedroom and I noticed a piece of paper on my pillow. It was a typed and printed-out letter from my dad. It was short, and explained that he couldn't live with Mom anymore, and that they were getting a divorce. This is when the tears started to pour. Alan read the note, a look of disbelief still on his face. He had also received a note on his pillow. I'll forever be appreciative that he sat me down to share the news, rather than leaving me to find the letter. Thinking about it now, it must have been terrible for him to have to be the one to tell me.

I was stunned that my parents were splitting up, that my family was falling apart, and even at twelve I knew this was not something you said in a note. Eventually my mother came home, crushed. We learned that our father had moved in with our grandpa. Dad came over the next day to talk to us in person. He picked us up in his old two-door pickup truck. Since I was the youngest and smallest I always had to sit behind the passenger seat in those tiny, fold-down seats. It was January and there was snow on the ground, and the sky and everything around me, and within me, was gray. We drove around in his truck, and I don't remember anything from that conversation. I only remember crying hard and that my nose was running like crazy. And I didn't have any tissues.

From that moment on my love and friendship with my brother only grew. As little kids we tolerated each other, but after this moment we learned how to truly lean on each other. There were many late-night chats and tears over our parents splitting up. How were we going to handle all of these unexpected changes in our lives? What were holidays, birthdays, and graduations going to be like now? Looking back, I am so grateful that Alan was there for me. I needed him, even though he was just a kid too.

After that we saw Dad on weekends, and every Monday night he drove Alan and me to the Rod & Gun Club (for a long time I sincerely thought it was called the Rotten Gun Club) for fly-tying lessons. This was an unlikely hobby that I picked up, mostly because my father and brother LOVED fishing, and I LOVED them enough to tag along. After a few lessons I did end up enjoying it, mostly because I liked working with my hands and all the glittery ribbons that were involved in the process. I had my own small vise and tackle box that was filled with metal hooks, thread, and all different colored furs and glittery ribbons that were used to make the flies, or fishing lures. The idea was to make the hook look exactly like a fly, or a small fish that the bigger fish would love to eat. This was also around the same time I got into jewelry making, so my tackle box filled with colorful beads and string sat right next to my tackle box full of fly-tying materials under my twin-size bed. This was also one of the Lovewell siblings' first adventures as entrepreneurs. We got pretty good at making flies and figured out a way to sell them to the local bait and tackle shop for money.

One Monday evening when my dad picked us up at the house, he handed us each a small bundle wrapped in foil. "I thought you two might want these cookies." Cookies? I felt my heart drop and before I knew what was happening, I burst into tears. "You don't know how to make cookies! Who made these? You have a girlfriend, don't you? Tell me where these came from!" Dad was angry at me for being so dramatic. From his perspective, he was just trying to give us cookies. But for me, it was like he had inserted a stranger right into our lives.

My intuition was right, of course. A couple of weeks later we would learn that my father had left my mom for another woman. It was a crushing blow to all of us, and I was furious with my father. I couldn't believe my dad could love someone else. Why didn't he want to be with us anymore? The anger I felt toward my father was a heavy weight I carried for a long time.

The next few years of my life were marked by huge adjustments. My world as I knew it had shifted. It wasn't just that Dad didn't live with us; it was that my mother was truly suffering, and this was taking a toll on me and my brother. She was heartbroken and felt alone in a community where there were virtually no other Asian people. To make matters worse, like many teenage girls, I wasn't getting along with my mother. Alan had gone to college, and the two of us were left alone in a house full of tension. We fought constantly about everything. Our behavior toward each other was dysfunctional; we were competitive, hostile, and unsupportive. We both had a lot of work to do on ourselves, and when my mom started dating, things only got worse. She'd be elated at the start of a new relationship and then heartbroken again after a seemingly promising relationship ended. I felt like my mom was totally checked out and that I was on my own. Then I went to a routine doctor appointment and discovered I needed her more than ever.

When you visit a gynecologist for the first time in your late teens you don't expect to be told you have a lump in your breast. I thought I was young and healthy, but now I was terrified that wasn't the case. On the Vineyard, there was just one doctor to whom I could be referred to investigate further, and she only worked on Wednesdays. I set my alarm so I could call her office first thing. I couldn't stand the idea of waiting an entire week to know whether it was something serious. I was scared and alone, and it somehow felt wrong to be scheduling an appointment with a specialist by myself. I was just a kid! I shouldn't have to do this! The doctor was able to fit me in that day. She examined the lump. "I'm not worried about this, but you should have it removed." Facing surgery, even a minor one, was not something I could navigate on my own, but I also knew that my mother was not in a place where she could help me. I didn't know what else to do. So, I called my dad. My anger toward my father remained a complicated ball of emotions. I loved him so much, but he had ripped apart our family and it still hurt. Could I depend on someone who had hurt me so much? Could I even let myself feel vulnerable and ask for help from someone who had caused so much pain? But I needed support, and I needed him.

Dad took me to the doctor's office the day of the procedure. I was told I couldn't wear contacts, and when I took off my glasses and couldn't see, I felt scared. The surgery went by quickly, and everything was fine, just like the doctor had assured me it would be. But I was completely disoriented when I woke up. The doctor apparently showed me how to change the gauze on my dressing, but I was so out of it that on the way home I was surprised to find a roll of gauze in my hand. "What is this?" Dad laughed a little. "Emma, don't you remember when the doctor showed you how to change the bandages?" I shrugged; I had no memory of it. "Let's get you home. Your friends have food waiting for you." The mention of my friends waiting for me at home reminded me that my mom wasn't. During those years she was coming and going a lot, and we were more like roommates whose busy schedules occasionally collided. Dad walked me to the front door and hugged me gingerly, not wanting to hurt my incision. I was so glad I'd called him, that I'd let go of my anger for long enough to let him help me. He got me through that crisis moment, and it was the beginning of a thaw that would bring us to a new place.

Over the next couple of years, we would discover two more lumps, two more benign tumors to be removed (thankfully I haven't had this problem in my adult years). My dad was by my side for all of it. Going through this kind of health crisis helped me discover a lot of things I hadn't known about my dad, like that he felt strongly that young people should be educated about sex and have access to the healthcare they needed to stay safe. He drove friends of mine to Planned Parenthood, never asking questions. This was a quiet way for him to show he cared. My dad is also my biggest advocate for many things, but especially for writing. Not long after my dad left, I decided to write him a heartfelt and also mean handwritten letter on a piece of pale-yellow lined paper. I wanted him to know what a crappy father he was and how he had ruined all of our lives. After he read it he said, "Wow, Emma, you're a fantastic writer." Which is possibly the worst thing I could have heard when I was trying my hardest to be cruel. He has always encouraged me to write and often gifted me journals for my birthdays. I believe it's because my father is a fantastic writer himself, and I think he always hoped that I would take after him. When I told him I was thinking about writing this book he almost exploded with excitement over the phone and then immediately sent me twenty books on "how to write a book."

As I mentioned, my dad always said that "anyone can be a storyteller," and his skill at spinning a good yarn is definitely one of the things I came to appreciate about him back then (but especially now!). When I got a bit stuck while writing a section of this book, I reached out to him for a little encouragement to break through the writer's block. What I got back was this incredible list of tips for telling a great story. Not only did it "unstick me," but I thought I would share them with you too!

FIVE TIPS FOR STORYTELLING INSPIRED BY MARK ALAN
   LOVEWELL, EMMA'S DAD

1. *GET THE AUDIENCE'S ATTENTION FIRST*

Make sure you have their undivided attention before you
start. Whether it is a small group of friends or a large audi-
torium, make sure you have the audience's attention, otherwise you'll lose them really fast. And noisy people, they'll
likely spoil the listening pleasure of those seated nearby.
They are annoying. Before you speak, wait until everyone
has stopped talking and they are looking at you. You might
throw a word out there that you are waiting. As a last-ditch
effort, you can call out to the guy in the back of the room.
Shout, "Hey you. Can you hear me?" When the guy says yes
or no, come back with a lightning-speed response: "Well, I
can hear you." Bottom line, you can't tell a story if people
are not listening.

2. *KNOW WHAT YOU'RE GOING TO TALK ABOUT*

Have an idea of what you are going to talk about! Every
story has a beginning, a middle, and an end. You don't
have to know all three parts before you start, but you
have to be prepared to tell a story that takes a person
through those three parts. It helps to have a hook,
something that is relevant and connects the audience
to the story in a personal way. The middle can feature

the adventure. And last, wrap it all up. What ultimately happens?

3. BE FRIENDLY AND CONNECT

You can even be self-effacing to grab their interest. But be kind. You must always be charged with lifting an audience. And there has to be something that connects them to the story, so make it relevant. If it is a rainy day, weave in a rainy day. There has to be glue that connects us all together. For the audience, storytelling is mostly listening to ourselves, as the storyteller weaves together their story.

4. INCLUDE A SPECIAL DETAIL

Include some deliberate detail that only a listening audience can connect to. This is not a shopping list of storytelling pictures and images with a cornucopia of facts. Just share one detail that might carry you forward with your story. It is an anchor. It is a human sense: sound, color, temperature. Pick something that you and your audience can call up in the story today and tomorrow.

5. GATHER TOGETHER

There is a shortage of fellowship between humans these days. And we are all trying to make it through a host of travails, a host of troubles. Wouldn't it be fun if storytellers gathered together to share experiences and swap stories? We could all use more positivity in our lives.

Every time I think about how my dad sent me those tips to inspire my writing it makes me so happy that I didn't let my anger at him dominate the relationship we grew to have. I had to tamp it down to reach out for help with my medical situation, but because I did, my dad was able to be present for me for all of those hospital trips, and it really shifted something in our relationship. I still carried some resentment, and I missed being a unit of four, but now I knew that my dad would always be there for me. He might not be at the table for Christmas dinner (and this hurt), but I could count on him for love and support the way I always had. We were no longer a tight-knit clan living under the same shingled roof, but our love for each other didn't have to change.

UNCONDITIONAL LOVE DOESN'T EQUAL PERFECTION

At first, I was reluctant to lean on my dad, because I was letting his decision to divorce my mother define *our* relationship. I believed that he could abandon me too, and I put up a tough front. I will never fully understand what happened to my parents' relationship; maybe they grew apart or fell out of love, but the dissolution of their marriage didn't have to mean the destruction of the family I loved if we both didn't want it to. Life is short, time is precious, and perspective is everything. I started to look at both of my parents with a different lens, and I made peace with their imperfections, embracing them as inextricable parts of the whole person I loved. I know they always embraced mine. I could love them with all my heart without expecting them to be perfect.

We can love people unconditionally—spouses, partners, friends, children, parents, grandparents—but that doesn't mean we won't face periods of disappointment from them. Unconditional love doesn't require perfection. My father is nurturing, creative, and kind, and those qualities didn't vanish with my parents' divorce. Once I replaced judgment with compassion, our relationship improved. I couldn't control what happened in my parents' relationship, but I could control how I chose to move forward with my relationship with each of them. Forgiveness is freedom. I forgave my dad, realizing it's not possible for me to understand what he was going through. I forgave my mom too; her life had been torn apart and she was doing the best she could to heal. She didn't have any support, and for the first time in her life she was focusing on herself. She was in therapy, she was dating (for the first time! She had only ever dated my father!), she was thinking about her work, a new career. I was independent and she trusted me. So I had a lot of freedom. I learned to appreciate both of my parents for who they are as individuals. They weren't together anymore, but I could still have a sing-along with my dad, and garden side by side with my mom for hours. I embraced their flaws, and I love them both for the unique gifts they bring to my life.

FORGIVENESS IS AN ONGOING PROCESS

The words "I forgive you" are not a magic pill. I believe forgiveness is the first big step toward repairing a relationship and letting it blossom anew. Forgiveness isn't about being "okay" with whatever happened. You aren't giving anyone a free pass to hurt you. It's a process that requires acknowledging what happened, being clear about your feelings, and making the bold decision to leave the moment behind as you move forward. I have forgiven my parents, but that doesn't mean all my emotions surrounding that period of my life disappeared as easily as a popped bubble. The pain isn't as acute, but I have trust issues from all this that creep in on occasion. I can be skeptical of other people, questioning their motivation. *Is this a real email inviting me to speak at an event? Or is this spam, or maybe a scam?* No one reads more online reviews than I do. Before buying almost anything, I read every review, trying to ensure I won't get ripped off. While some of this is just being smart, I'm aware I take it to an extreme. Who does an hour of research before buying a lipstick? Sometimes I must check myself—is there something to this, or am I being cautious because I'm afraid of being hurt again? I realize there is a little seed of mistrust left inside me, and I have to be mindful that it doesn't take over. When I sense this happening, I take a moment to acknowledge it. Feel the fear and then move forward anyway. I lean to skepticism, so I know trusting people is sometimes an act of rebellion. I like to reflect on positive moments with each of my parents as well. Making dumplings with my mother, listening to my father's never-ending supply of interesting stories. These are the kinds of gifts they are continually giving me, and it helps to remind me that I am loved.

Forgiveness can be scary, and it's hard to leave past hurts in the past. Remember that this process is *about you,* the forgiver. Anger is a very heavy burden to carry, and the longer you hold on to it the more damage it can cause. Anger can hurt relationships, your self-esteem, your mental health, and your well-being. Don't give all your energy to a past hurt. Let it go and see how the open space in your heart fills up with light. As I look at the sparkling night sky on the Vineyard, I remember how loved I felt watching a meteor shower in the middle of the night in my pajamas with my dad. I felt safe and protected, and like nothing could ever change that. My life did change, but those feelings about my dad didn't need to change along with it. The night sky on the Vineyard is always spectacular, endless spots of brilliance against a black sky. But that's not all that's going on: 275 million stars are born and die each day. The same sky I marveled at with my dad is living and dying every second. Stars themselves can be gone in a flash; it's *the change* that's constant. Not every change is welcome; some hurt like hell. But like an old star reaching its end, that hurt will start to fade and eventually it will be gone. Let it go.

FIVE

Being Thirsty Can Make You Stronger

Walk around New York City for five minutes and you'll see that diversity is on full display—everywhere. People move here from far-flung places all over the globe, and there's a comfort to seeing faces of every color. Here, being different because of my mixed-race heritage makes me fit right in. I'm just one of many. Growing up on the Vineyard I felt self-conscious about being Chinese. There weren't a lot of people who looked like me, and it was undeniable that culturally we were "different" in my house. As far as I knew, none of the other mothers had meditation pillows or Buddha statues on full display in the living room. None of my friends ever mentioned having fermented vegetables for dinner or hot pot for a celebration. Those same things that made me feel like our family was weird—meditation, gardening, fixing things—those became the foundation of a balanced life and a successful career. The journey to embracing who I was at my core took years, and when I think about this period of my life it makes me realize the growth that can happen when you release the struggle to be like everyone else and recognize *you are enough*.

Every day in the school cafeteria I felt like my differences were on display for everyone to see. I would open my lunch box with equal parts fear and anticipation. I always enjoyed what my mom packed me for lunch, but the truth was, being the only kid with a bento box full of traditional Chinese food could be embarrassing. My lunch was the polar opposite of what was contained in the Hello Kitty and Spider-Man lunch boxes of my peers. As I opened the box each day, the heads at my lunch table turned toward me, wondering, *What freaky food does Emma have today?* "Emma, what is that? A rotten egg? Why is it all brown and white? *Gross*. And is that a pile of dirt on your rice? Are you actually going to eat dirt?" I looked at my lunch, a tea egg, rice with rousong (also known as meat floss), and pickled vegetables—all foods I liked to eat, lovingly made from scratch by my mother. Tea eggs were a favorite of mine. They're soft-boiled eggs cracked just slightly, then boiled again in a mixture of tea, star anise, and soy sauce, which makes them look like big marbles (sometimes they are called marbled eggs). I knew how delicious the egg would taste and I wanted to eat it right away, but I felt too self-conscious. Powdered pork (a dried meat that's a light and fluffy topping for things like rice and tofu) was another common food in my house, but something about the fluorescent light of the cafeteria made it look like it was from outer space. Sitting there surrounded by Wonder Bread sandwiches and individual bags of neon-orange Cheetos, I wished I could transform my lunch into something more "normal." As I picked up my chopsticks, I knew my bento box and I stuck out like sore thumbs.

When a friend stayed for dinner, I felt a flush of anxiety before we sat at the table. I knew my mom's cooking was delicious, but I never knew how a friend would react when they realized dinner at my house wasn't going to be meatloaf or spaghetti and meatballs. When my friend Amanda stayed for dinner, I was happy to see that she didn't balk at the Chinese dishes my mother had set out. She looked intrigued. Amanda dug right in. "Wow, this is really good." She was happily chewing away when suddenly her face turned bright red. She started coughing and her eyes were watering like crazy. Then came the sweat, pouring right down her now inflamed face. "Amanda, are you okay?" She nodded awkwardly, waving her hand in front of her face like she had a mouthful of fire. Which, essentially, she did. A bell went off in my head, *ding ding ding*. I knew exactly what had happened. "Oh, no! Amanda! Did you eat one of the dried hot peppers?" Her face just got redder. "Mom, Amanda ate one of the dried peppers!" Mom rushed around getting her a cold glass of milk and a plain bowl of white rice, anything to quell the heat. The dried peppers were supposed to flavor the dish but weren't meant to be eaten. I had never actually eaten one, because I had been warned that they are hotter than the surface of the sun. Pushing those peppers off to the side was second nature to me, but it didn't occur to me to warn Amanda. Amanda's face turned back to its normal color soon enough, and she was a good sport about it. But I felt so embarrassed that this had happened. *Things like this wouldn't happen if we ate spaghetti and meatballs like other people! No one ever set their mouth on fire eating meatloaf!*

While my Asian-inspired meals made me feel like the odd one out on the island, there were just as many times when I did not feel Asian *enough*. My mom is the youngest of six siblings. She's also the only sibling who married a white person. All my cousins were raised in Chinese households, with two Chinese-speaking parents. They grew up in Asian communities where things like hot pot and tea eggs were normal and taking Mandarin lessons was a given. Two times a year we'd all gather at my aunt and uncle's house in New York, where I felt like just as much of an outsider as I did on our predominantly white island. While there was just one generation separating me and my grandmother, in many ways it felt like we were born centuries apart. She didn't speak English, and I only knew a few words and phrases of Mandarin. Other than me waving, giving her a big smile, and saying, "Ní hǎo," we couldn't communicate. The typical granddaughter/grandmother conversations like *You've grown so much! Why don't you come see me more?* or *I hope you're being good to your mother and getting good grades at school* didn't exist between us. Our mutual acknowledgment of and respect for each other was the extent of our connection. Having respect for elders is a huge part of the Chinese culture. There is no lack of respect in our family, especially toward my grandma Po Po. She just turned 106 years old and has seen more in this world than anyone else I know. She has lived through multiple wars and civil wars, and immigrated to many countries. She lost her husband in a tragic train accident and had to raise six children all by herself. She may be only four-foot-nine, but what she lacks in height she gains in resilience and toughness, and she will beat anyone at a game of mahjong. She still doesn't understand what I do for a living, but I honor her and love her nonetheless. The rest of my cousins, who took Mandarin classes and spoke the language at home, could have real conversations with Po Po, while I stood back feeling like a visitor. My cousins would do their best to fill me in on what everyone was saying, but sometimes I'd let myself sink into the background, remaining quiet and imagining what the conversation was about.

I am aware that I can pass as white, but when we went to New York, my looks suddenly set me very far apart, especially when we went out for dinner. We'd go to a Chinese restaurant that was frequented almost exclusively by Chinese people, always sitting at a table big enough to fit the entire clan. There was lots of laughing and dozens of Chinese dishes ordered: crispy noodles, garlic soy steamed whole fish, scallion pancakes, and fluffy pork buns. The waiter moved around the table filling glasses of water and passing out chopsticks. As soon as he reached me and Alan though, he abruptly stopped and turned around. I knew exactly where he was going and what he was doing. When he appeared again a few seconds later, he was holding two forks—one for each of the white kids. I looked at the fork like it was a snake that had popped out of nowhere, a potentially dangerous thing separating me from the rest of my family. I looked at Alan as if I were saying *Don't worry, I got this*. I looked at the waiter and said, "Yoǔ kuài zi ma?" a turn of phrase I'd mastered specifically to avoid this embarrassing situation. Looking surprised, he quickly removed our forks and handed over the chopsticks, which Alan and I had been eating with since we were old enough to chew. I was always keen to enjoy the huge spread of food my relatives ordered, but my inability to blend in often made it hard to feel like I belonged at that table.

Not belonging was a constant tension in my life, and I pictured it almost like a taut rubber band. On one side was my white family, the relatives on my father's side who had lived on Martha's Vineyard forever. They had history there. On the other was my mother's family from Shanghai, by way of Taiwan, steeped in their Chinese culture even though they had set down roots in America. I bounced back and forth between each. I was constantly trying to find my footing between the two cultures, whether I was explaining, *No, that's not a rotten egg,* or I was smiling as big as I could, trying to show my grandmother respect and love with just a facial expression. There always seemed to be a reminder that I wasn't enough of either.

I struggled with my cultural identity for most of my life, and a big piece of that was curiosity about my mother's homeland, which I had never visited. I followed in my older brother's footsteps in college and studied abroad in Beijing. It was a challenging and exciting experience, and I connected so much with what my Chinese heritage meant to me, but I wanted to experience Taiwan through my mom's eyes, to see the land that had shaped her into the woman she became. In 2018 we finally planned a family trip—me, my mom, Alan, my baby nephew, Luca, and my sister-in-law, Jenn, who was actually the catalyst for this trip. She's super adventurous and very good at organizing and was so excited about taking her son to see his grandma's homeland with all of us. One of our first stops was the Taroko Gorge on the northeastern coast, a huge twelve-mile canyon with fairy-tale-level beauty. Its cool, smooth marble walls shoot hundreds of feet into the sky like majestic ivory towers, with the Liwu River winding through them down below. The white stone contrasts beautifully with the aquamarine water. Our next stop was a surfing town. Most people don't associate Taiwan with palm trees, black sandy beaches, clear water, and tropical fruits, but the northern half of Taiwan is subtropical, and the southern half is straight-up tropical and hot. I felt like I was in Hawaii. Alan is an excellent surfer, and I've spent years trying to catch up to his skill level. Like a typical older brother, he taught me to surf the hard way, throwing me right into the ocean in Santa Cruz, California, known for its ultra-challenging surfing conditions (that's a story for later). It was humbling, but I survived. After that Alan and I took his dream vacation and traveled to Bali, Indonesia, to go surfing for a month. We stayed in four-dollar-a-night accommodations and went surfing every morning and every sunset. It was in Bali where I finally felt confident surfing in the water. Physical activities and extreme sports have always been a bond between Alan and me. After long days of surfing on those Taiwanese beaches, Alan, Jenn, and I would buy cold coconuts and pork buns and talk for hours, everything so warm and tropical it was easy to forget we weren't on the California coast but in Taiwan, the place of our mother's childhood.

In Taichung, we popped by one of the Peloton factories. My mother's eyes lit up when she saw the big sign featuring a picture of me that said, "Welcome, Emma and family!" As the elder of our family, my mother was treated like royalty on this visit, everyone fussing over her and making sure she, a queen, had everything she needed. She was so happy and inherently so proud of me. The general sentiment in Chinese/Taiwanese culture is *If it wasn't for your mom, you wouldn't be here, Emma.* This is why honoring and respecting your elders is such a huge part of the culture. Something was shifting in me. For so long I didn't feel Chinese enough, but if it wasn't for my mother, if it wasn't for the beautiful country we were visiting, if it wasn't for her courage to leave for America and conquer the hardships she faced as she settled in New York, I wouldn't be here. Without my Chinese mother there would be no me, and while I was "only half" Chinese, my roots, really, had started growing here, in Taiwan, my mother's homeland.

The last thing we did on the trip was visit the neighborhood where my mother was born. My mother grew up in an apartment complex and was very poor. Her building no longer existed and had been replaced by a park. Mom started pointing out where things used to be, "This is where we lived; this is where we played outside." Suddenly she got quiet. "I can't remember the Taiwanese word for subway." She had been in America long enough that parts of her native language were no longer available to her. She snapped her fingers like the elusive word was at the tip of her tongue, but she never found it. Mom continued walking around the park. "It's nice to be back; I think I'd like to retire here." She looked happy, and I understood that my mother's life was also measured in two parts. Coming back to Taiwan all these years later, she was now more American. But at home on the Vineyard, even after living there for decades, she was still more Chinese. Like me, her existence stretched like a rubber band between those two poles.

At our last family meal in Taiwan, my little nephew was

like a tiny ambassador of joy, spreading love with his smiles and being fawned over in restaurants as he gobbled up everything from dumplings and pieces of watercress to jackfruit and fermented vegetables. I looked at my nephew, working on a dumpling with his chubby hands. My mother sat next to her first grandchild with a contented smile on her face. At that table three generations of a family were bonding over the simple deliciousness of a dumpling. After years of being the lone tea egg at a table of peanut butter and jelly on one side and the girl whose handiest Mandarin phrase was "I'd like chopsticks, please" on the other, I felt at peace. I had viewed being half-Chinese as a problem that needed to be solved, but it turns out having a foot in two different worlds was what bonded my family together. I left Taiwan with a deeper sense of connection to both. And if I had to ask for chopsticks at restaurants for the rest of my life? That would be okay.

THIRSTY ROOTS CAN MAKE YOU STRONGER

If you plant something in the ground and it doesn't rain for a while, the plant doesn't always die. Many times, it adapts. Not having what they need sometimes forces roots to grow deeper and spread farther until they hit the water they need to survive. I dealt with my own kind of thirst for years. I was thirsty to fit in on the island and thirsty to feel accepted by my mother's family. I'm not sure what my life would look like right now if I hadn't had to stretch and grow to quench that thirst. I might not have studied abroad in China when I was in college; I might not have set down new roots in a city where practically everyone is from somewhere else. Searching for my identity led me to be curious about Chinese cooking and growing my own food, which has brought me closer to my mother and enhanced my connection to our culture. The questioning and desire to understand where I fit in pushed me to seek out answers about where I came from. I am stronger, happier, and comfortable in my skin because of this exploration. The self-reflection, stretching, and growing were hard at times, but once I finally hit that water, drinking it in was even sweeter. Self-reflection is a powerful tool. When you explore who you are, many things come to light along the way. Your perceptions change; you'll experience breakthroughs and see how capable you are. If you keep the process moving forward and commit to learning about yourself, eventually you will find what you need to nourish yourself.

For years I wanted to feel acknowledged and included, accepted for who I was. Thinking I had to be one thing in my dad's world and another thing in my mother's just kept me off balance. I didn't feel like I had strong footing in either place. It took a long time to understand that there was no need to try to be two places at once. There weren't two halves of me; I was a *whole person*, comprised of different backgrounds with unique talents and her own perspective—and she was more than enough. It is freeing to realize you can't control the perceptions of others, I couldn't snap my fingers and make myself more Chinese or all white—and, more important, I didn't want to. My roots had grown and stretched, and by the time I hit that water I knew one important thing. I'm enough, and I always will be. Embrace your differences, celebrate your quirks, and don't change to match someone else's perception of how you should be. Because you are already enough just the way you are.

SIX

Don't Be the Queen of Difficult Things

If you've ever procrastinated, then we have something in common. I've built a career around fitness, but the truth is *I don't always feel like working out*. I am a master of excuses. I'm too sore; I'm tired; I haven't spent enough time with Dave lately; I haven't spent enough time with the cats, gardening, or organizing my extensive collection of leggings. There's also the universal *I don't feel like it* that can spread through all aspects of your life like a bad rash.

In my life now, I know that when I hear that negativity from my inner voice, it's a signal to change my mindset. I quickly flip my thinking from *But I don't want to* and instead say, "I'm going to take this opportunity." But for a long time, I wasted energy being mired in negativity of my own making. It took time, but I learned how to release myself from self-made difficulties by changing my thinking, tapping into my passions, and surrounding myself with interesting and supportive people.

This next story is a little embarrassing. Believe it or not, there was a time in my life when I acted like an entitled brat, whining and complaining about everything as if the world owed me a golden ticket to happiness. I was eighteen years old and I was leaving Martha's Vineyard for college. When I look back at myself during that time, I cringe. I was kicking and screaming (just metaphorically) the entire way because I didn't want to go to the University of Massachusetts at Amherst. I actually believed going to a state school was a tragedy of epic proportions. I had my entire life ahead of me but arrived on my college campus with a huge attitude because I thought I deserved "better." I had trapped myself in a cage made of ultra-negative thinking and self-pity, and it almost kept me locked up, nearly ruining an amazing moment of growth and opportunity.

I did *everything* in high school. I got good grades, even in my AP and honors classes. I played piano for the mandatory thirty minutes a day, I was captain of the soccer team and the lacrosse team, I took dance classes and was in the company at my dance studio, participated in the annual musical theater play every winter, and was a singer in my high school's choir, the Minnesingers. Our performance of Handel's *Messiah* "Hallelujah" in the annual Christmas show at the Old Whaling Church was *legendary*.

I held down multiple jobs while doing all that. Tourism is a huge industry for Vineyarders. There was a downside (traffic, entitled vacationers, "washashores" aka people who moved to the island but weren't actually *from* the island). But the upside was plenty of opportunity to make money while hanging out with my friends. When summer came along, I was 100 percent hustle. I worked as a lifeguard on South Beach during the day, my nose covered in zinc oxide as I stood on the guard stand blowing the air horn at swimmers who were pushing their limits. At night I bartended or waitressed at the Sand Bar or Balance, shaking up rum punches and pouring countless glasses of rosé for vacationers and summer folks who had spent the day out on their yachts. After many hours of saving swimmers and/or mixing stiff drinks, I still had enough energy to party with friends late into the night. Most of my friends had jobs as well, and there was always an after-work house party, usually in someone's parents' garage apartment or basement. After a fun night with friends, I was still able to get up early and do it all again.

I was busy 24/7, all year round, and because I pulled it all off with good grades and a good attitude, I wanted "more" for myself than a state school. I am mortified to say this— but I thought UMass was the place where the kids in my high school who *didn't try* ended up. I was obnoxious enough to think that because I had *sooooo much* to offer, scholarships to "the Best Schools" should have fallen out of the sky and landed on my doorstep. I sent out my college applications to many private and out-of-state schools even though I knew my parents could not help with any of my tuition. "Go ahead and apply anywhere, Emma, but just keep in mind that you have to pay for it." My summer income of bartending and lifeguarding was not going to cover the costs of those schools. Most of my friends had parents who were able to offer at least some financial support. They could mostly go to any school they got into. This did not wear well on me. I was jealous, and self-pity was seeping out of my pores. State school was the most practical and affordable option, but I hated the idea of practical and affordable. I was so sick of those two dull adjectives in reference to my life. Didn't I deserve impractical and expensive? Growing up around the wealth on Martha's Vineyard, I saw how the options for families with money were different. I resented the fact that I had worked so hard but didn't have the same options other kids had. Looking back on it now, the root of my brattiness was all because of disappointment, a disappointment that the things I'd been told about meritocracy and "hard work" weren't really true. It was the first time I realized that you couldn't necessarily get whatever you wanted just by working hard. I didn't know then what I know now: People with money do have systemic advantages, and no amount of busting my butt was going to overcome all of them. It was a hard and lingering truth to learn. It came across as brattiness, but it stemmed from a real reckoning with how the world is.

The thought *Why can't something good happen to me?* ran through my head on repeat like a reverse mantra. I didn't know it, but I was making everything worse *for myself*. I landed on the campus of the University of Massachusetts at Amherst with a chip on my shoulder the size of the island I grew up on. I never even visited the campus before the day I moved in. I let that giant chip weigh down my entire early experience of college.

For the first time in my life, I was facing a big challenge and I hadn't prepared. The amount of research I did about my new school was ZERO. In a lame act of rebellion, I didn't sign up for any activities. What's the point of getting involved? I'd participated in loads of activities in high school, and where did that get me? This "shitty state school," that's where. I hadn't investigated any of the majors, telling myself it didn't matter which classes I took. I was phoning it all in. I went to class, did my work, turned in my papers, and studied for exams, but there was no joy to be found in any of this. I was putting in the work to get decent grades so I'd eventually *get that degree*, but I wasn't even trying to have a meaningful experience. I slogged through each day cloaked in anger and bitterness. I was the self-anointed Queen of Difficult Things who spread her unique brand of misery everywhere she went.

When I didn't immediately connect with other students (probably because of my bad attitude), I took it as another sign that I was in the wrong place. It was disorienting. In my fantasy world, college was an enchanted place where I would make unbreakable, lifelong bonds with like-minded people. I thought that within five minutes of landing on campus I'd fall in with a group of people and know *these are my future bridesmaids!* But surprise, surprise . . . it didn't happen. As my first lackluster and lonely semester creeped forward, I finally mustered up the courage to audition for the choir. I didn't make the cut. I took this disappointment as proof positive that my life sucked. I halfheartedly researched the soccer teams and intramural sports but never got myself to show up. I considered pledging the Asian sorority, but as a mixed-race woman I worried that I wasn't Asian *enough*.

As Queen of Difficult Things, I managed to convince myself that nothing was within my control. My unhappiness was solely the fault of this stupid school. My experience would have been the opposite if I had gone anywhere else. I would have been tapped to be in a secret society that met in a renovated dungeon. I'd be debating other students while sitting on a lush plot of green grass, the fall leaves gently blowing around us. And my dorm room would surely have a fireplace and a window seat. But this delusion wasn't reality. I would have to force myself to slog through until it was time to limp across the stage at graduation to get my dumb diploma. I could picture it now, in a cheap frame that I'd probably keep in the back of my closet under a pair of rusty ice skates.

Emma Lovewell
Summa Cum Laude
Bachelor of Arts in Bratty Behavior with a
Concentration in Self-Pity

Out of desperation, I considered taking a dance class. There were two types of dance classes at school: the classes for everyone and the classes for dance majors that required an audition. Hmmm, an audition? I noticed I felt a little tingly thinking about that. It was a familiar feeling. *Oh! This feeling is excitement. I forgot how this felt while living my difficult queendom.* It also tapped into my competitive side, which had been lying dormant since I left the island. I started practicing dance moves in my dorm room to prepare. I showed up to the audition and gave it my all. Every hair flip, pas de bourrée, and pirouette was done full out and *with feeling.* I made the cut. Dancing in college wasn't going to solve all my problems, but it felt good to have finally experienced a success. I was meeting other dancers, learning new choreography, getting exercise, and feeling the joy that comes with moving my body to music. More important, though, I was letting some sunshine in. The forecast for my day-to-day existence changed from cloudy with heavy rain to partly cloudy with a chance of sunshine. I had a ways to go, but it was an improvement, and feeling warmth on my shoulders was wonderful. Reengaging with something I loved, *regardless of where I was doing it,* was the thing that finally pulled me out of the trap I'd built for myself and set me on a welcome new path.

My interest in dance and the arts inspired me to apply for internships. And a few semesters later, I landed two dance-related internships for college credit in New York City. I was a marketing intern for the avant-garde theater PS 122 and worked for an all-female hip hop dance company called Decadence. It shouldn't have been a surprise that I fell head over heels in love with New York City. Growing up, I'd sit in the back seat during the long ride from Massachusetts to New York, so excited that I'd get a stomachache. By the time we hit the city it was usually early in the evening, and I'd be bouncing up and down in my seat, in awe of how the lights made everything feel so big and bright. The energy of the city was so strong it felt tangible.

After our arrival at my aunt and uncle's house, we'd eat a big dinner, and I'd sit at the table trying to follow along in the conversation, which was strictly in Mandarin. Although my mom's family didn't show affection through words or hugs, I always felt love through their generosity and the many meals that we had together. The next day we set off on our usual New York City routine. My mom (who lives for a good bargain) loved the fourteen-dollar haircuts we could get in Flushing. I'd walk in with my regular hair and walk out freshly snipped and flatiron straight. We'd visit the Asian grocery store to stock up on foods we couldn't get on the island. After filling the cart with bamboo in hot oil, pickled mustard greens, spicy instant noodles, frozen dumpling wrappers, and all the vegetables and fruit we could fit in the car, we'd hit another site on the tourist to-do list. Our trip would end with dinner in the Village at my uncle's restaurant Wok & Roll. After eating his secret, off-the-menu dishes that we got as VIP customers, we'd head back home. I'd watch the city get smaller, already looking forward to our next trip.

Unsurprisingly, I suppose, my experience as a newly minted adult in the city was quite different from my childhood visits. I hadn't seen anything like PS 122 in Queens. PS 122 is a performance space that was started in 1980 in the *pre*-pre-gentrified East Village. A group of artists took over an abandoned public school (PS = public school/performance space), and the scrappy, raw space became a place where New Yorkers went to see groundbreaking, avant-garde theater, music, visual art, dance, poetry and prose readings, and film. While the bulk of my job was to rummage through magazines searching for reviews and press write-ups, I was also getting an education observing every person I encountered there. I marveled at their drive, creativity, and curiosity. People came to perform in this space from all over the world. Art was their passion; it wasn't something they just did on the side. I saw that it was possible to build a life around what you really love, but it required effort.

My fascination with New York City life extended outside of work too. I had found my apartment in classic New York City fashion—a-friend-of-a-friend-of-a-guy-I-dated-knew-a-guy whose roommate was away for a few months, and did I want to live in their room in Brooklyn? The apartment was small, dingy, and next to the Brooklyn-Queens Expressway, but everyone who came through the door had a dream they were pursuing with purpose. I didn't want to be the sad-girl-who-does-nothing anymore. I wanted a dream too. I wasn't sure what the dream was, but I knew *this* was where I wanted to be when I figured it out. When my internships were over, I went back to school to finish my degree, but this time I had focus. Graduating would mean getting to come back here, to a place where I could be surrounded by interesting people and tap into the electrifying energy of city life.

When I was stuck in the role of the Queen of Difficult Things, I was a drag of massive proportions. I didn't seek to find a bright side, ensuring my life was full of negativity, boredom, and loneliness. I refused to open myself up to anything, kicking and screaming that college was *such a bummer*. I had trapped myself in a cage of my own making, and I didn't understand that I was the one with the key. We all face our own storms, but sometimes they're products of our own creation. If you started the storm, you also have the power to stop it. The bad attitude I cloaked myself in in college guaranteed that the experience would be as horrible as I'd imagined it would be. I had written THIS SUCKS across my forehead *in Sharpie*. I wasn't willing to let anything in or anyone chip away at the wall I'd built around myself because it would mean admitting that my preconceived notions were wrong, bratty, and just plain crummy. But here's the thing about being a self-anointed Queen of Difficult Things: It's not that hard to knock yourself off that throne. Unlike with real-life monarchies, it doesn't take a full-fledged war to strip yourself of that crown. In retrospect, I am so grateful I had that experience at UMass. My parents were right in teaching me a meaningful lesson. I got a great education, and it was one I could figure out how to pay for on my own. Learning to navigate a huge university having grown up on a small island was a feat in itself. The experience of going to college and having to pay for it put me in an amazing position for life after college.

LET YOUR PASSIONS LEAD THE WAY

Sometimes, one change is all it takes to let some light shine through. For me, it was auditioning for dance classes. Arriving in the studio each day reminded me, finally, that *there were things I enjoyed*. Dancing was a way to shake off some of my attitude and let some joy back in. Whenever I catch myself complaining, I remind myself that I have the power to take control. I'll start by engaging in an activity I'm passionate about (dancing, gardening, exercise, yoga, biking, and cooking are all on my list). Doing something you love helps you focus on the present while leaving any other stresses behind. Immersing yourself in a hobby keeps you engaged mentally and physically, and it's often a pathway to making social connections. When you make room for the things you love in your life, your days get easier and your life gets brighter.

Find Your People

Connecting with like-minded people or with people who encourage you to grow can be a huge motivator. Meeting people with big dreams and lofty goals inspired me to want more for myself. The energy and curiosity I encountered in New York City was contagious. I wanted to be part of this new and interesting world, and that wasn't going to happen if I was withering away in my prison of pity. I saw what freedom could look like: making new friends, learning new things, and having new experiences. Being in the company of fascinating people pushed me to become the best version of myself, and I don't think there are goals more worthy than that. While it was hard to be faced with the prospect of connecting with a new group of people in college and when I moved to New York City, all I had to do was look at a photograph from one of the "fake weddings" my closest friends and I planned over our summers on the Vineyard throughout college to be reminded that the effort is worth it. Parties on the Vineyard are shut down regularly by the police, but Martha's Vineyard is one of the top wedding destinations in the country, and *weddings rarely get shut down.* My Vineyard crew and I saw an opportunity here. We realized if we couldn't have a party, we *could* have a wedding. We organized a potluck, rented tables, decorated with flowers, baked a cake from a box, and even had our friend's band set up and play. We decided who our lucky couple would be, and after two of our friends pretended to get married, we enjoyed the rest of the party without any concern that the police would shut us down. In this particular picture my friends and I are beaming. We are having fun, but I like to think those smiles are about something bigger. We banded together to make something unique and silly happen. We were making memories and strengthening the bonds that already held us together. It can be so hard to build new friend-ships as an adult. It takes time to find the people we really click with. But when I look at the picture of my girlfriends in their fake wedding finery, I'm reminded that when you find your people, the ones who understand you, provide unwaver-ing support, and will even pretend to be bridesmaids so your party won't get shut down . . . it's a huge gift.

Explore an Unfamiliar Place

I love to travel, and there is nothing like placing yourself in a completely unfamiliar environment to urge you out of a self-imposed dark spot. Traveling forces us to be flexible when navigating new environments and promotes empathy. Inter-acting with other cultures or people we don't know adds a big dose of novelty to our lives. When we learn about others we become more appreciative of our differences. It's not even necessary to travel, just go somewhere new. Pushing yourself to try a different coffee shop, restaurant, or gym shakes things up. An unfamiliar space can be inspiring and uplifting, and it puts you in a position to meet new people and try different things.

My time as the Queen of Difficult Things did not serve me. Sitting on my throne, judging everyone and everything, just ensured that I would stay trapped in that dark, drafty old castle. Exploring passions and opening myself up to a big city and different people showed me there's an entirely new queendom out there that I'd like to conquer. And I couldn't wait to see what life would be like in a whole new realm.

SEVEN

You Can Change the Energy of Any Room You Walk Into

I have always believed that dance is one of the most satisfying forms of fitness because it's fun and also good for your body *and your soul*. So, it's probably not surprising that launching the Dance Cardio program at Peloton with my teammates has been one of my professional highlights. The launch of the first set of classes was a big success, especially with people locked down in their homes, missing the dance floors and flashing lights of nightclubs. Ally and I were asked to program more classes for cardio, and the request this time was that we'd be choreographing a new all-Usher Dance Cardio workout, one that was going to have a surprising twist. We practiced some of our favorite hip hop moves, rehearsing a routine that wasn't too hard to follow but would get everyone's heart pumping. Ally and I spent hours in the studio perfecting our moves. Ally is not only a fantastic and talented dancer but she's also one of my closest friends. When the two of us get onto the dance floor together, we are quite literally unstoppable, and the fun and positive energy is palpable. We were having so much fun practicing this dance that it was hard to remember that this was work!

The day of the shoot we were ready, and I was buzzing with excitement. The surprise bonus for this workout was that Usher was actually going to dance with us. I was going to dance with one of my teenage idols! This was a major "how did I end up here?" moment. Dancing with Usher was simply not in the realm of possibility during my early years in the city, and now I was *collaborating* with him? It felt unreal.

When I was a young dancer trying to land jobs, the hustle was nonstop, and it was hard. I didn't really know the direction my life would go, but I was positive that I wanted to stay in New York and that it would take every ounce of creativity to figure out how. Staying meant taking crazy jobs, regularly working until dawn, and worrying each month if I was going to make enough money to pay my rent or buy groceries. It was a challenging time, but I learned that if I brought my best energy to every experience, I could transform each crazy job into something positive. Coincidentally, a few of my current colleagues at Peloton were in similar situations as I was at that time. Ally, Cody, Jess King, Rebecca, and Hannah Corbin were dancers I'd see often at auditions, and I booked jobs with most of them at some point in our dance careers. One ongoing gig in particular still makes me smile when I think about it. Cody and I had jobs as backup dancers for a pop singer who was big with the LGBTQ+ crowd. For months we'd go to gay nightclubs to perform with this singer, always covered in body glitter and enough hairspray to suit an '80s glam rock band. That was our ten minutes of fame. We'd perform the three to four tracks, whipping our hair and body rolling to the beat, as people in the crowd would yell and cheer for us. If you don't know Cody, he's hilarious, and if you do know him, then you know Cody was always Cody-ing. I felt like such a rockstar diva on that stage with him, and I always left those jobs incredibly sweaty, laughing my ass off the whole way home.

I have been working since the very minute I was legally allowed to. My parents had always told me there was much wisdom to be gained from hard work, and I was excited to join the ranks of the employed the moment that anyone on the Vineyard would hire me. This mindset prepared me well for New York City, because if I wanted to stay, I had to be prepared to take almost any money-paying gig that came my way. In retrospect, I have to say I've had some very, um . . . interesting jobs. But I set my mind to learn something from every one of them, and to view each one as a step on the way to wherever I was headed.

When I first landed in the city, many brands and artists were expressing their creativity by hiring people to be involved in "experiential marketing." These experiences were definitely a trend, and they became an unexpected source of income for me. One memorable event that comes to mind was going to a party/performance in Williamsburg, Brooklyn (this area, at the time, was ground zero for hipness). I was in a big open room with fifty party guests and fifteen secret "actors." It looked like a normal party, stylish people standing around with drinks and talking to one another. I was chatting with a party guest, and he was telling me about the true crime documentary he was producing. I was about to ask him a question when I heard the distinct but subtle cue. I watched the documentarian's face change as I started to speak AS LOUDLY AS I POSSIBLY COULD WITHOUT SCREAMING. I kept a straight face and acted normal even though the volume of my voice was at its maximum. My fellow actors were all doing the same thing. With half the people in the room talking loudly, it was a real cacophony. Just as quickly as the loud talking started, it ended. I acted as if nothing strange had happened and asked the producer (who was not a secret actor) in my regular voice, "What initially drew you to the topic of your documentary?" He opened his mouth to answer just as I heard the next cue.

I began dancing rhythmically, purposefully, and then broke into larger movements, taking up more of the space. I was not holding back, really going for it, moving all over the room. The guests' expressions quickly turned from a collective WTF? to amusement, to joy, as they absorbed the "experience" around them. This "experience" was the work of the site-specific choreographer Noémie Lafrance. She creates large-scale pieces and often uses the architecture of New York City as a background for her work. She's the artist who choreographed a dance piece in an empty fifty-thousand-square-foot pool in Brooklyn, and the one in the twelve-story stairwell of a parking garage. The gig I did with her was some seriously high-level artsy stuff, and I was into it.

THE TAKEAWAY: Don't do half-crazy. If you're going to do something that's out of the box, go for it. Don't hold back.

Flash mobs (remember those?) were a popular way to advertise in my early years in New York, and they became another . . . interesting way to make money. For one flash mob I was sent to Washington, D.C. It was the middle of the day and I was standing on a busy street that was packed with pubs, bars, and restaurants. If anyone noticed me, I looked like a regular woman who was out grabbing a coffee or maybe meeting a friend for lunch. Suddenly a huge party bike (picture a bar on wheels) pulled up. If you hadn't noticed ten people pedaling a bicycle that was the size of a small-town tavern, the loud music that started up would have gotten your attention. The hyped-up pedalers leapt off the bike flashing Mr./Ms. America smiles as they offered free cups of light beer to the residents of our nation's capital. Then it was my turn to take action. I moved toward some other bystanders who were actually dancers. We formed a circle, and then I burst out of it with some fancy footwork, launching into my most badass break dance moves in the middle of the street. People were staring, some were clapping, many were confused, some were chugging down their free beer, while others were visibly annoyed. Once it was clear we had made an impression by disrupting everything for everyone (and giving out free beer), the cyclists hopped back onto the giant bike and we made our way to the next location, where we'd do this all over again.

THE TAKEAWAY: Being paid to dance feels amazing, even when it's dancing in the middle of the street giving away light beer.

In 2012, I landed the one-off gig of a lifetime. Backup dancer for the Rolling Stones. Is there anything cooler? Before the concert began, the dancers who had been hired for the show were each holding a pair of drumsticks and strategically hidden in the many wings/aisles leading into the stadium. We had rehearsed many times and were prepared and so excited. There we were, standing in a stadium full of people, ready for the show to start. I remember looking up into the audience and seeing Sarah Jessica Parker, and then Johnny Depp walked by. Then the band played the opening chords of "Get Off of My Cloud," and we emerged from the masses and started banging our drumsticks on chairs and railings, slowly making our way onto the stage in front of an audience of nineteen thousand people, where we danced for the opening song.

THE TAKEAWAY: A few bursts of well-placed enthusiasm have the power to fill a huge space with positive energy.

Then there were all the music videos. Some of these were so bad that I'm not going to say what they were because I still want you to respect me. I will share that one video was shot in a McMansion in New Jersey, where the dancers could only be filmed from the knees up because the owner was worried about his marble floors and wouldn't let us wear shoes. I was in a Latin music video where I played a woman who cheats on her boyfriend at a nightclub. Think telenovela. The casting director thought I was Latina and assumed I could speak Spanish (I'm not and, alas, I can't). That gig was awkward.

I *will* share that I was in the Björk video for "Declare Independence." This video was directed by Michel Gondry, who also directed the film *Eternal Sunshine of the Spotless Mind*. I'm one of the people in a helmet jumping up and down while Björk shouts at us through a megaphone. Just try to spot me.

THE TAKEAWAY: Sometimes you have a take a job to pay the bills. As long as it doesn't compromise your values, go for it. You never know where it will lead.

Cobbling together enough random jobs to survive was rough, and I was exhausted by the constant hustle. So, when the agency that booked my gigs called to see if I was available "right now" to audition for a two-month dance gig, I threw on sweats, a tie-dyed tank top, and my high tops, and raced out the door. When I arrived at the audition space there were already a few dancers practicing a combination. A woman who had an "I'm in charge" vibe started waving frantically at me. "Who are you?" she shouted over the loud music. I shouted back, "I'm Emma Lovewell. You called me a half an hour ago?" She just nodded and pointed to the women who were dancing, indicating I should join in. They were dancing to a classic rock song, and I fell into step effortlessly. We easily fed off each other's energy and we were perfectly in synch. A few seconds later the music abruptly stopped. "Okay! That was great, ladies. You're all in. We leave in two weeks and rehearsals start right now. I need you for the next four hours at least." A smile spread over my face, because hurray, I got the job! And a two-month-long gig? That sounded like heaven compared to all the one-off jobs I was doing. But also, *we are leaving for where exactly? And to do what?* The confusion must have showed on my face because In Charge Lady said, "Well. Do you wanna be in the circus or not? I don't have all day here!" *Circus?* I admit I wasn't expecting that. "Oh. Yes! Definitely. I'm in."

I wondered what I had just agreed to. As visions of elephants, trapezes, and people being fired out of cannons flashed through my head, I noticed a woman in baggy sweats and a cropped tank had just walked into the room. We were about the same age, and we clearly shared similar ideas about what to wear to auditions. In Charge Lady shouted, "Thanks for coming, but I've got everyone I need." The woman gave a quick sigh of frustration and then just turned and walked out, her graceful gait proof positive she was a dancer too. There was something about watching her leave that pulled on my heartstrings. I imagined that, like me, she had gotten the call at the last minute and had also dropped everything to get here as quickly as she could. Our situations could have easily been reversed if my train had been late or if I couldn't have found clean sweats in my laundry quickly enough. In this city, just a couple of minutes can make a life-changing difference. I knew that part of the reason I got the job was because I got there first. Her time was wasted, and after going to dozens of auditions I knew what it felt like to feel dispensable. This time I had the good fortune to be on the right side of the equation.

And that, ladies and gentlemen, is how I ended up spending two crazy-magical months of my life touring with the Most Interesting Show in the World sponsored by Dos Equis. Oh, and it wasn't technically a circus, it was a *variety show*.

The first thing I'd hear upon waking up in the morning was the doves cooing from the back of the tour bus. I'd pull back the curtain of my sleeping cubicle and get out to stretch. While sleeping in a space the approximate size of a coffin sounds terrifying, I usually fell asleep as soon as my head hit the pillow. There was something about the wheels of the bus on the rolling highway that lulled me into a slumber. The dancers were housed toward the front of the bus. The performers who required live creatures for their acts were in the back near the cages of doves and the aquarium full of scorpions. I didn't let myself think about being in a confined space with those scorpions, which are, apparently, so predatory that in addition to eating bugs and spiders, they'll happily dine on each other. We'd occasionally hear, "Hey! There's a Petco a couple miles off the next exit! I need to stop and get a new scorpion!" shouted nonchalantly from the back of the bus.

Following a big morning stretch and a glass of water, I'd look out the window to see the landscape as we flew along the highway. After a few hours of spotting truck stops, fast food restaurants, fields of corn, fields of nothing, churches, and the occasional Bates-style motel, this wild cast of characters would pull up in another college town. We'd get decked out in our costumes, ready to perform our show, which was a wild mix of dance, burlesque, and vaudevillian antics.

The music would start and I'd be all dressed up in a red sequined corset. I held a huge fan and had enough feathers on my person to pass for a Las Vegas showgirl. I'd slide out dramatically onto a stage. The sound of applause and hearty cheers made my soul light right up. I was with four other identically dressed ladies. We opened the circus with a sassy dance number, using our sparkle and shine to prime the audience for the show they were about to see. This show included: a man balancing a running lawnmower on his head while a woman threw cabbages at the lawnmower blade, a singing burlesque performer who wrote on people with lipstick, a magician and his doves, a husband-and-wife team who shot crossbows at each other, and a pair of contortionist twins. The act involving scorpions isn't something I care to recount. I was cast as a dancer, but I was also a makeshift magician's assistant, handing over weapons and cabbages to performers during their acts. The purpose of all this was to promote Dos Equis beer, whose commercials at the time featured "the Most Interesting Man in the World." Sometimes the actor who played this role would make an appearance, and the audience would corner us after the show and ask, "Tell me, who is he? Was he in the military? Is he from out west? He's gotta be a spy, right?" I'd nod my head politely, never having the heart to break the news that the man they were inquiring about was a fictional character.

The circus was a free show with free beer, and the young people who came to the performance were all in an extraordinarily good mood as a result. Every night the vibe was so positive it was like we were continually arriving on the last day of exams. After the performance we'd all be buzzing from the charge of energy. The generosity was next level.

People treated us like rock stars, so grateful and appreciative, asking for pictures, wanting to talk with us. Sometimes people would let out a happy scream and reach out to touch our hands like they were at a Rihanna concert. As someone who has bartended at countless bar mitzvahs, I can tell you this was preferrable to being screamed at by a pack of thirteen-year-olds who were waiting for their Red Bull.

The fun went on for hours, and at times it felt like we weren't just plying people with free beer, *we were spreading joy*. The thrill of performing and getting a big response was all encompassing, and as soon as one of these nights ended, I couldn't wait for the next one to begin. After a cocktail or two we'd all retreat to our bus as our normal selves—stripping off feathers and makeup and other equally outrageous outfits. Meals were microwaved, teeth were brushed (I once famously brushed mine with beer when we ran out of water), scorpions were fed, and we'd all get settled, fall asleep, and wake up in a new city to do it all over again. We performed in more than fifteen cities. It was a fabulous way to see the country. The companionship I felt as we pulled onto the highway each night, ready to sleep en route to a new destination, was as comforting as a feather duvet. We were like a well-functioning family. Each person had their own unique energy that contributed to the fun.

YOU CAN CHANGE THE ENERGY OF ANY ROOM YOU WALK INTO

I didn't immediately see the magic that was happening while I was doing whatever it took to set down roots in New York City. I thought all the hustle was nothing more than a necessary series of stepping stones. Earn money, pay my dues, pay my rent, REPEAT, and hope it all added up to something. But taken collectively, these jobs and experiences showed me that I wasn't just doing a job. I was directly contributing to the energy around me.

Energy is extremely contagious, and you have the power to impact the energy anywhere you go. On a basic level you can use your smile and positivity to light up and inspire smiles or stomp around like a storm cloud that's about to pelt everyone with cold, unrelenting rain. I could have viewed each job as a hurdle to jump over to get paid. While earning money was essential, I *chose* to bring everything I had. I made a pact with myself. If I was taking *any* job to help make ends meet, I would bring the best of me to that job. I could face another bartending shift dreading how much my feet would hurt, or I could decide, "Maybe I can break my record of making forty vodka tonics in under three minutes." I took as much pride in my bartending work as I did in my dance gigs. If you view something you need to do as a slog, it's going to feel like a slog. When you think of a task as an opportunity to be more efficient, more precise, or more engaged, your spirits will be high, and time will go by faster.

I might have played a small role at the Rolling Stones concert, but I wasn't *just dancing*. I was contributing to the level of excitement in that huge space. When I was in the variety show, each performer had a specific role. When those talents were combined it turned into something bigger. I wasn't a lone dancer in sequins and feathers. The lawnmower guy wasn't an oddity to watch while you threw back a beer. Collectively our contributions created a magical experience that held everyone's attention.

It's similar at Peloton. My teammates support each other. When Ally and I put together a Dance Cardio routine or a Two-for-One Ride, we are feeding off each other as we bring you an experience that energizes and inspires you. If we are having fun together that energy will transfer to you in your living room.

All my jobs, whether I was dancing or pouring drinks, contributed to this important change in my mindset. That I do have control over my environment, that I can shift the energy of a room. I have never rushed into the Peloton studio last minute and hopped on the bike. That's baseline, that's the minimum. As I'm getting ready to go live, I'm thinking, how can I make this ride inspiring for healthcare workers who are exhausted? How can I make this a great experience for new moms who barely have time to breathe? What can I do to inspire someone to get back on the bike again tomorrow? It's always *What can I share with you?* These little moments are where differences are made. It's where we transform something good into something excellent. It's where we find pride and accomplishment from the mundane. It's where we trade in mere completion for a goal-crushing success. Energy is the difference between just okay and WOW. And the source of that energy is you. Tap into it, use it, and change the vibe of every room you walk into.

EIGHT

Yes Is the Antidote to Regret

When Dave and I arrived in San Pedro, Chile, we were already at an elevation of eight thousand feet. Traveling to Chile together had been on our bucket list for quite a while, and it felt like a dream come true when we arrived. We were excited to explore but knew we had to take things slowly so our bodies could acclimate. We spent the first day hiking along a river in the middle of a desert, surrounded by magnificent giant cacti that were hundreds of years old. We had never seen anything like them. The next day we were ready to take things a bit higher and went mountain biking. As we made our way up to fourteen thousand feet it was difficult to breathe, but we took it as a challenge. Other than the car that followed us for safety, we didn't see a single person. As I was pedaling, I saw a mass of pink out of the corner of my eye. When I realized what I was looking at I could barely believe it: "Dave, those are flamingos!" It was crazy to see flamingos in the wild, and at higher points we saw vicuñas and guanacos just wandering around on the mountain. But not even the wildlife we saw on the way up could compete with the view at the top. Long stretches of mountains and deserts, capped with a never-ending sky.

On our last day we hiked to our highest elevation yet, climbing all the way up to eighteen thousand feet. To give you an idea of how insanely high that is, Burj Khalifa in Dubai, the tallest building *in the entire world,* tops off at 2,717 feet. At eighteen thousand feet the oxygen levels drop to 52 percent, and that can be very dangerous, so we took things slowly and carefully. My body could feel the difference in oxygen levels with every step I took. This hike wasn't easy, but it was worth it. When we reached the top, we were rewarded with a magical 360-degree view. We were so high up we could see Bolivia and Argentina in the distance! After growing up on an island at basically sea level, I felt like I had landed on another planet. I marveled at the view, but as I stood at what felt like the top of the world, I also thought about how I got there. I wouldn't have had this fantastic, once-in-a-lifetime experience if I hadn't mustered up the courage to use one word—YES. It sounds so simple, but the change you can create by just saying yes can be life-altering.

As I was building my career as a fitness coach, I learned that if I wanted to have a following, I'd have to push myself right out of my comfort zone. That meant diving into social media and learning to be open with strangers. I had to post pictures of myself and share my thoughts, which wasn't easy for me (you might not believe this, but as I mentioned in my lip-synching chronicles, I'm naturally private and introverted in real life!). I forced myself to network and meet new people in the fitness industry. I pushed myself to say yes to doing things before I felt ready for them, like posting recipes even though I wasn't a chef or making videos for my social media when I didn't completely know what I was doing. And although I knew being in the public eye would open me up for scrutiny and judgment, I knew I wanted to take the risk. Saying yes is operating out of abundance and optimism, not scarcity and fear. Writing this book is another example of saying yes, and although it is terrifying, here we are (please be kind). The trip to Chile was the result of a connection I'd made on social media after years of gathering followers. I could never have imagined the first time I posted on @emmalovewell that I would be collaborating with a travel company in the middle of the Andes mountains. Those first tentative posts helped pave the way for much bigger things later on.

As a fitness coach, I see how saying yes to small things leads to big results over time. Committing to the Crush Your Core program is like saying yes to being stronger. Eating vegetables with every meal is saying yes to a healthier body and digestive system! Of course, exercise and nutrition won't bring instant results, but over time the small changes can add up to something significant. Saying yes often means a leap of faith, because we can't always forecast what the results will be. I understand the desire to know how a choice might impact you down the road, but sometimes it's in the unknown where we find some of life's biggest wins. Magical things can happen when you say yes and open yourself up to new possibilities.

One of the many risky Craigslist ads that I responded to was for a gig as a model for a personal trainer's website. The ad was looking for a female athlete who was comfortable at the gym and willing to show their stomach and abs. It paid fifty dollars. But I responded anyway, thinking maybe it would pay for a nice dinner! I ended up booking the gig and showed up to the set in the photographer's apartment in Long Island City. Luckily the job was legit, and the personal trainer and the photographer were kind and professional. This shoot ended up changing my life.

The photographer was Jay Sullivan, the same photographer who shot the cover of this very book (life really does come full circle sometimes). He was mostly a lifestyle and headshot photographer at the time, but as we started talking he admitted that he was trying to get more into fitness photography. He noticed that the fitness industry was really taking off and that there were tons of brands looking for fitness photos, from publications like *Women's Health, Fitness Magazine,* and *Men's Journal* to fitness and fashion brands like Tory Burch, Under Armour, and Athleta. I told him I was trained as a dancer, and he said to me, "Have you ever thought about being a model?" I thought, *Me? Really?* While I have plenty of confidence in my appearance, in a million years I would never have imagined myself as a model.

But when I thought more about it, I realized that, as a dancer, I already felt comfortable onstage and in front of a camera, and knew that I took direction well. I had those skills. I also knew I was always filled with judgment when I would see an ad for a major brand with a "dancer" leaping in the photo with the same arm and leg forward, and a sickled foot. I would always shake my head and think, "Wow, they should have hired a *real* dancer for that shoot." I listened to Jay's words and took them very seriously. *Yes, I should give this a try.*

Jay invited me to come back to do a test shoot so we could create images for my first-ever portfolio. I showed up a few weeks later to Long Island City at five in the morning so we could shoot during the warm light of sunrise. Running along the boardwalk next to the water, and then stopping out of breath and sweaty, looking off into the distance: These were all "fitness-y" moves that I learned that day. These photos got printed on nine-by-eleven-inch photo paper at Adorama and then placed into the leather portfolio with my name emblazoned on it that I had purchased from the House of Portfolios.

I got signed by Wilhelmina Models within their fitness division (and ended up working with them for seven years). It was one of the most significant things that ever happened to me and really launched me into the fitness community in New York City. In just a few weeks with the agency, I was flying around the country doing photoshoots for Athleta and Under Armour, where I learned the minutiae of the job, like how to turn the left side of my abdomen a fraction of an inch so the photographer could get the most muscle definition for the shot. I made connections with brands, I learned about how the business works, and for the first time I felt confident that there was success in my future, even if I didn't know exactly what that looked like. I was starting to believe my world would consist of more than a long string of low-paying jobs; I could almost see an end to the hustle and stress. And in 2012, I did a Kickstarter commercial shoot for a fitness start-up company called Peloton. I did the job in a day, acting as a home rider who took a class on their new at-home stationary bike. The premise was "hop on your bike at home and then get completely transported into a live energetic in-studio class." I had no idea how important this shoot would be someday.

That yes to a fifty-dollar Craigslist ad led me to enormous opportunities. It's eventually what landed me where I am today. While it would be years (and many more jobs) before I would join the Peloton team as a cycling instructor, I was finally seeing how all the different parts of me could potentially fit together into a career where I would thrive.

The next and crucial piece came when I made a promise to myself that I would stop bartending and find a career that highlighted my strengths by the time I was twenty-eight. Just six months before that crucial birthday I got a call from a friend. "Emma, so I've been teaching cycling classes at this studio. They're looking for new people, and by the way, they offer health insurance." That was the YES moment that led to my very first job as a cycling instructor . . . promise to self—kept!

LEAVE NO ROOM FOR REGRET

Not too long ago I was really feeling myself on the bike while teaching an EDM ride. I felt the beat in every part of my being; I felt light, positive, happy, and free. There are times when I spend hours preparing what I will say during a ride, but honestly, most of the time I give myself space to let the motivation come to me. With the right song, during the right moment, I am able to listen to myself and say what I know I need to hear in that moment. That's my secret to motivating you: being open enough to myself to know what I need to hear and then trusting that maybe you need it too. At this point in the ride, I had a lightbulb moment. What if we put an end to all those times when we wished we had gotten out on the dance floor? We should say yes more often so that we never wonder, *What if?* I believe we regret not doing more often than we regret doing. The experiences that come from saying yes can be so meaningful, whether they change your life or bring you a single memorable moment. When I'm on the Vineyard and my dad and brother want to take me fishing, my first reaction is a big groan because that means getting up at three A.M. I'd rather be sleeping, but saying yes to fishing means spending time on the sand with two of the people I love the most. The stars will be amazing, I might catch a huge fish, and my dad and I might have a wonderful conversation. Those are moments I don't want to miss. Fishing may not alter the course of my life, but that doesn't make the experience any less special.

Getting out on the dance floor of life isn't about being perfect either. There are gifts to be found in failure too. Years ago, I had an audition for a gig that required tap dancing. This was a style of dance I had minimal experience with, but I didn't want to let that stop me. I decided I would learn the steps and do my best. I was feeling confident and figured, why not? I had my hair in a high pony and was wearing what I thought were adorable, albeit very tight, red denim shorts. I moved through the choreographer's first few steps easily enough, but I struggled with the high kick at the end. My shorts were so tight that I could barely kick my leg at all. I decided I would hold back a bit while we were practicing and then go all in during the actual audition. When it was my turn, I gave my ponytail a tug and got into position. I was in the middle between two other dancers. The music started and I was really holding my own considering tap wasn't my thing. When it was time for the high kick, I whipped my right leg into the air as hard as I could. But my denim was so restrictive that when it met the force of my kick, I went flying. The music came to a stop at exactly the same time my body hit the ground. I was lying on the floor while I heard a collective GASP from every single person in the room. The women on either side of me stuck their arms crisply into the air for the final pose. "Oh, my God. Are you okay?" the choreographer asked, looking genuinely concerned, but also like he might laugh. I forced myself up quickly and nothing seemed to be injured (aside from my spirit).

I was horribly embarrassed, but I learned an important lesson that day. There are times when saying yes doesn't lead to a personal victory or even a positive outcome. It's about joining in, doing your best, seeing where it all leads, and, most important, having no regrets. When you say yes, you open yourself up to a future full of meaning, because life's most significant moments, big and small, come from those times when we force ourselves out of our comfort zone. Each yes might not always end the way you imagined it, but that doesn't matter. You showed up and you gave it your all. So, try new things, take risks, and dance more! Even if you fall flat on your face. You are a player in this game; you're not supposed to only stand on the sidelines.

THE COURAGE TO SAY YES: A PRIMER INSPIRED BY KIMCHI

Like many New Yorkers, my partner Dave and I decided to leave the city during the pandemic. There was so much uncertainty, and the city was packed so tightly with people. I don't need to tell you what a difficult time that was, and I am so grateful that I am here and healthy. After moving through a few temporary outposts, we had the good fortune to be able to rent a small house on a lake upstate. I know it was a huge blessing to have our own outdoor space and to be able to keep a safe distance from others. I've always loved the water, and I got in the habit of taking my paddleboard out every morning. There is something so peaceful about gliding around the sun-kissed water in the quiet of the morning. And because my cat, Kimchi, who was born in an alleyway in Queens, is a bold and adventurous cat, I'd let him out to roam for a while, since for the time being at least, he was a country cat. This was a big change for him; until recently, his entire world consisted of a tiny one-bedroom apartment in the city.

Every day he'd sit on the dock, not budging at all as he watched me move around the lake. All summer long it was like this. One morning in the fall, as the leaves were all turning a brilliant yellow, I got onto my board, and Kimchi walked all the way out to the end of the dock. I decided to paddle up in front of him to say hi, and he surprised me by leaping onto my board. I was shocked and equally thrilled! I gave him a few seconds to adjust. Once it was clear he was staying put and not going to leap off the paddleboard in fear, we floated around together. I have to admit, I assumed it was a fluke—a one-off cat adventure. But apparently Kimchi didn't get the memo that cats and water usually don't mix. The next morning, he joined me on the lake again, and nearly every morning after that. It's like once he took that first leap of faith, he was all in. Taking a leap of faith is hard, but here's hoping we can all learn something from Kimchi, the paddleboarding feline.

STEP ONE: ACKNOWLEDGE AND CONFRONT YOUR FEAR

New things are scary. If they weren't, trying something new wouldn't be such a big deal, but it also wouldn't be so exciting. Facing something unfamiliar can be terrifying, but that's okay. Tell your fear that you're aware of its presence, but you're not going to let it hold you back.

STEP TWO: GET COMFORTABLE WITH DISCOMFORT

Accept that it's possible that you might experience discomfort at first. Just lean into it, and now your discomfort will likely be temporary. The mix of uncertainty and anxiety you're feeling right now? It's actually an opportunity to learn, grow, and progress. The feeling will pass.

STEP THREE: DON'T LOOK BACK

This is your "jumping onto the paddleboard" moment. You've made your decision, you've accepted it's scary—now just go. Keep in mind that the fear of trying something new is often more intense than actually doing it! Just. Let. Go.

STEP FOUR: TAP INTO YOUR NEW SOURCE OF STRENGTH

You took the leap and you survived. You might have just learned, aerial yoga is NOT for me, or wow, aerial yoga, where have you been all my life? Whatever the end result, you've given yourself a real gift. You know now without a doubt that you have the courage to try new things. Tap into the memory of this moment whenever you need it. And remember, Kimchi is always there for you, rooting you on and urging you to jump off that dock!

NINE

If You Focus on Scarcity, You'll Always Feel Lacking

When Dave and I we were getting ready to close on our house I was in full-fledged operating mode. There were so many ducks to line up and the paperwork felt never-ending. I was equal parts excited and nervous. *Am I actually buying a house? Can I really make this work?* The truth is, for a long time I couldn't have imagined that home ownership would be in the cards for me. I thought buying a home was for other people who had more money than I did. When I signed my name for the last time and was handed a key to *our house,* I couldn't believe it. I looked at the single key in my hand, thinking, *This tiny object has the power to open a great new chapter in my life.* I told myself, *Remember what this moment feels like. You worked so hard to get here!* As I stood in the kitchen that we planned to rip out and renovate,

I took a deep breath. I had evolved so much since I was that struggling young woman who was building a life and a career, having no idea if it would lead anywhere. It was an exciting phase in my life, and I was grateful for this more solid ground I had reached. As I looked out the sliding glass door to our backyard, I remembered how worn down I used to feel when I thought about everything I didn't have. I don't think I'm the first person who wondered if the hard work would ever add up to something. It's so easy to get caught up in the view of what we don't have that we often don't notice what's right in front of us. That's why I want to talk about how life becomes fuller and more satisfying when you stop focusing on scarcity.

I was sitting on the bus with my fellow circus performers on another long stretch of highway when I decided to check my bank balance. It's not something I enjoyed doing, because this was back when money was a constant source of stress. After I paid my rent and bills and bought a subway pass and groceries I would often have just a few dollars left. I would try to tell myself, *Emma, you have what you need*, but this mantra didn't provide much comfort. I wanted something much more than the basics; I wanted security. The idea of waking up every morning knowing that there was enough money to get through sounded like a luxury. I couldn't imagine what it would feel like to work hard at a job without panicking about what was next. I know anyone who has worked as a freelancer might have felt this same way. This is a small thing, but some days I wanted to splurge on a Starbucks coffee without worrying I wouldn't be able to pay for something essential . . . like soap or toothpaste. When it came to money it felt like there were two directly opposing versions of me. There was the positive version of Emma, who hustled hard and did whatever it took to make ends meet, while the negative side couldn't stop stressing about the precariousness of her own life. Negative Emma would also be envious of anyone who wasn't one missed gig away from paying their rent.

Since we were driving through the middle of nowhere, it took a while for my bank information to upload. When it did my jaw just about hit the sticky floor of the bus.

Checking Balance $2,745.42

I had been in the circus for only two weeks, and this was the most money I had made consistently since moving to New York. I was being paid $1,000 a week and getting a per diem for food. I was subletting my apartment in the city, and it turns out there is nothing to spend money on if you live on a bus. I was in the unique position of earning money while having zero expenses. The math was easy, but it was still nearly impossible for me to compute. I'd have $8,000 when the gig ended?! I sat back in my seat, the vibrations of the road like a gentle massage to my back. *Emma, you've done it, you've managed to earn some real cash!*

When the circus gig ended, the holidays were right around the corner. I knew my family didn't expect fancy things, but the idea that I could buy everyone better gifts than usual sent my Christmas spirit soaring. I bought my mother a massager, a sweater I thought she'd like, and art supplies. I bought fancy sneakers for my brother, and my dad's gift got an upgrade too. Dad is the guy who *wants* socks for Christmas. That year he got an extra-big supply, plus a few shirts and an extra-soft Christmas flannel for those brutal island winter winds. Christmas felt supremely merry that year. I was a full-fledged working performer who earned enough cash to treat my family to nice things for Christmas!

February arrived and reality hit me like a cold slap in the face. I wasn't booking new gigs and was relying solely on bartending for cash. I was short on next month's rent. I'm not proud of what I did next. I called my mother and asked her if I could borrow three hundred dollars. This was the first (and last) time as an adult I ever asked a parent for money. I had just given her elaborate Christmas presents when she would have been happy with anything, and now I needed to borrow money *from her*. The irony of the situation was not lost on me, nor did I feel good about asking my hardworking mother for help. My mother had always managed to make ends meet, so why was I having so much trouble?

I have had an awareness of money (or lack of it) since I was a little girl. My family's thriftiness wasn't limited to the home-grown vegetables on our table; my parents had to be careful about money all the time. Shopping for basics on Martha's Vineyard can be tricky. The Vineyard is known for beautiful beaches, spectacular sunsets, historic lighthouses, and delicious seafood. This is why the Vineyard is a popular vacation spot for celebrities and even former presidents. Walking along the streets of Edgartown with its fancy boutiques and quaint restaurants is like walking through a picture postcard. Notably missing are chain stores of any kind (the only exceptions are the Stop & Shop and the Dairy Queen, and let me tell you, when the Dairy Queen opens in March every year after its winter closure, every island kid is THRILLED and waits in a line out the door to get their Blizzard or dipped cone). This supports the local economy while simultaneously protecting the town's character and cuteness. But growing up as a year-rounder on an island where my family couldn't afford the more exclusive shops meant we had to be strategic about how and where we bought things. Every year before school started my brother and I were taken to the mainland to shop. This was our one opportunity to stock up on anything we might need for the year ahead.

"Emma, Alan! I need you in the car in five minutes! Or we'll miss the ferry." My mom didn't need to tell me twice. I always looked forward to our annual shopping trip to the mainland to visit the giant retail wonders that the rest of the country had easy access to. After we landed on the Cape we'd head straight for the Independence Mall, and we'd always start at Filene's Basement. The store was so much bigger than anything on the Vineyard that I would need a few minutes to adjust. I'd walk around gently touching everything, my head spinning. I had to examine my options carefully, since it was my only chance to buy things that were brand-new. If I outgrew my jeans during the school year, I'd be out of luck. I'd usually buy things a little big, so there was room to grow. The items I chose also needed to be affordable and practical, and I had to calculate the optimum fashion potential for anything I purchased. One year I fell madly in love with a pair of wide-leg pants on the sale rack at Limited Too. They were blue silk with a floral print. I twirled in front of the mirror. *I love these! But wait. Are these pants or pajamas? Do these look great, or do I look like I'm headed to a sleepover?* While I certainly wanted to push the cool-kid envelope when it came to clothes, it's hard to take risks when you're not seeing the mall again for an entire calendar year. My mom could tell I loved them. "Get them, Emma!" Those pants became my biggest shopping success story. I wore them on every special occasion (and not a single sleepover).

After buying clothes, sneakers, boots, socks, underwear, and school supplies, I'd usually buy a pair of earrings at Claire's and would pop into Spencer's Gifts to stare at the lava lamp for a few minutes. We'd wrap up our epic shopping trip with dinner at a chain restaurant like Friendly's. While I was eating my grilled cheese or chicken fingers, I'd glance at the card on the table advertising the clown sundae topped with a bright red cherry. On these special trips I was always allowed to order dessert. Our off-island dinner ended the same abrupt way every year. Mom would suddenly notice the time. "Kids, finish eating! The last ferry leaves in thirty minutes! Where is our waitress? We need the check! Finish eating! We need to be in the car now!" My brother and I would start wolfing down the remainders of our clown sundaes, washing them back with swigs of root beer from the largest cups we'd see all year. We'd fly out of the restaurant even though there was a good chance we'd just end up sitting in traffic on Route 28. Some years we flew out of the restaurant and made the ferry by a hair. When we missed it, we spent the night sleeping under scratchy sheets that smelled too strongly of bleach in the closest motel mom could find. I'd fall asleep stuffed into the tiny room with my family, knowing that the shopping bags lined up in our dingy space were filled with new things for a new year. Those annual shopping trips were full of hope and promise, school clothes, sneakers, leotards for dance class, fresh pencils, and Trapper Keepers and notebooks that would be filled with homework, dreams, and ideas. In those moments it didn't matter that we didn't have a lot of money; I knew I had everything I needed.

Unfortunately, as I got older, the feeling of joy and security I got from those shopping trips became harder to come by. It became difficult to be happy about what I *did* have because it was so easy to focus on what wasn't there. One night at my bartending gig in Manhattan I met a beautiful, dark-haired man named Brad with a killer smile who was pursuing his dream of being an actor. We'd chat at work, often staying for a late-night chat with my friend Katie. We were all in the same boat . . . big goals, few resources, and a strong will to keep that boat above water. I started to look forward to our conversations. Brad's dry sense of humor always put a smile on my face. Eventually, our work talks continued outside of work. We would grab something to eat or get a coffee and talk. Our conversations quickly evolved from the crazy things that happened at the bar to what we wanted to achieve in life. We both couldn't wait for that moment when we found a bit of success and could finally stop working in a bar. I loved that we were both hard workers and had bigger visions about what we wanted for ourselves. As we continued to get to know each other, Brad shared that he had battled drug addiction and was working hard to stay sober. I admired his openness and thought he was brave for taking the difficult step of working through his addiction. None of this scared me off; it made me respect him and like him even more.

We started dating, and Brad would become one of the most important people in my life over the next year and a half. He was so full of life that his presence allowed me to forget about my own struggles for a while. Brad was resourceful too. He'd take Katie and me out on the town, always to another restaurant where a friend worked so they could slip us some free drinks. After a couple of cocktails (and a Red

Bull for Brad), we'd all head home. As we walked to my apartment in the East Village, I'd look at all of the people packed into bars and restaurants, laughing with friends. "Do you guys think all of these happy people once worried about their futures as much as we do?" Katie put her arm around me. "Emma, we can't ever really know what's going on with someone. And why do you think success is an 'if'? Why don't you just think of it as a 'when'?" What she said to me that night was powerful. I started to push away thoughts of "if" and all the negativity that came along with them, and to focus on "when."

IF YOU FOCUS ON SCARCITY, YOU'LL ALWAYS FEEL LACKING

A scarcity mindset will drain the life out of you. I know what it feels like to worry about money and job security. It's scary, and I am so grateful I am no longer in that position. I do know that growing up without a financial cushion to rely on made me work even harder. While friends of mine would take big gambles, like starting companies or investing their money in new opportunities, I rarely did, because I knew if I failed there was no one there to catch me. So even though I would take some big risks with my career (it's not like moving to NYC to perform is ever a "safe" career choice, let's be real), everything I did was incredibly deliberate, and I always had a backup plan. This is something I still carry with me to this day. I still hustle and work hard, it never stops! When I think back to those early years, I was 100 percent focused on scarcity. Every day I was able to list everything I didn't have: security, a cushion, money for little extras. It was a long list. Scarcity was like a heavy weight I carried around with me at all times. It was all I could think about. Scarcity can take up so much mental space that you're not able to fully stretch and grow. The weight of longing and envy can become a huge obstacle in your quest to get what you really want. When you're operating with a scarcity mindset, it's like walking around with blinders on. You can only see the emptiness in front of you, there's no way for you to see any of the abundance and goodness right around you. Scarcity breeds doubt, putting us in an "if" rather than "when" mode of thinking. And if you don't put scarcity in its place, it will follow you around forever.

There wasn't a magical moment when I permanently switched from "if" to "when" thinking, but I know Katie's words had a great impact on me. I didn't know *when* success would arrive, but when I thought back to that scrappy little girl on Martha's Vineyard, thrilled by her fresh new notebooks, I realized I was proud of where she was right now. There were many unknowns, but I was making things work. I had found a new home, made new friends, and learned to navigate around a city that was bursting with energy and possibility. That girl *was* succeeding right now, even if there was much more she wanted to reach for. You can't suffer yourself to success. Take the blinders off and look around to see what's already there. When you acknowledge what you already have, you start to realize you have a lot. And being grateful for what you have is an incredibly powerful force that can create so much more positivity in your life. Abundance creates more abundance. What you focus on is what you get, so make sure you're focusing on abundance.

———

The day we finally got the keys, I walked into our new house through the sun-filled entryway. The space wasn't quite large enough to qualify as an actual room, and the walls were all lined with natural cedar wood panels. But as the light filtered through the window, I knew exactly how to transform this awkward, empty space into something special. I could envision a cozy wicker chair, big enough to curl up in with a cat and a cup of tea. I could imagine plants, lots of them, thriving in the bright light. I would build myself an indoor jungle. As visions of green plants blossomed in my mind, I thought about the last few years of my life. There was struggle and hardship, but I had finally learned to see the joy in the journey. I learned to view what I *did* have with gratitude and appreciation. I cherished my friends and family. I embraced the excitement in a city where I struggled to find a place to fit in. I stopped saying "if" and replaced it with "when." The unknown is scary, but it's worse to miss out on the good that's happening because you are so focused on the future. As I looked out that window from the space that would become my personal little retreat, I saw dozens of trees and rocks that needed to be removed to create a garden. We had a lot of work ahead of us, and it was going to be hard, but I wasn't intimidated. I knew we would have a spectacular garden, it was simply a matter of when.

TEN

Finding Quiet in a Noisy World

When my car is about fifteen minutes away from the studio, it's the perfect time to center myself before I arrive to teach a class. I sit up a bit straighter in the back seat as the driver tackles New York City traffic. I slowly start to breathe deeply, counting with each breath in and out. After a few minutes, the noise of the city is barely audible as I focus on the breath. When we pull up to the studio, I feel calm and prepared. I hop out of the car and usually smile for a few selfies with Peloton fans. Energized by these encounters, I know I can nail my rides.

Arriving at the studio in a rushed flurry sets the wrong tone for me, because I always want to be present for each ride. Even a short meditation can help me get into the right headspace. I know it feels like everyone is touting the benefits of a regular meditation practice these days, but there are good reasons meditation is becoming more mainstream. In a world that's overflowing with distractions, meditation is the greatest tool for stress management, improving your patience level, and ability to handle emotions with grace. Being grounded in the present increases your self-awareness, making it easier for you to see situations for what they really are. Meditation will not only de-stress you; as you'll see, it can also lead you down a path to a more positive and focused life.

I could say that I've been meditating since before I was born. When my parents were living in New York City in the seventies, my mom saw a flyer in Chinatown for a meditation lecture in a Buddhist temple in the Bronx. My mother fell in love with Zen meditation and is still a practicing Buddhist who meditates daily. She has gone on countless meditation retreats and went on silent retreats when she was pregnant with both me and my brother. I imagine her glowing from her pregnancy, existing in complete silence for those seven days with just me as I bounced around peacefully in amniotic fluid. I like to credit my ability to sit and breathe through my emotions to this in utero meditation experience. I grew up in a household where my mother regularly meditated. It wasn't unusual to walk into our quiet house looking for my mom and then realize she must be upstairs in her room meditating. Her practice is consistent: Every day she gives herself that time, sometimes just ten minutes, sometimes forty-five minutes.

My personal relationship with meditation didn't really start until I was about seven years old. One day I came home from school, grabbed a snack, and walked into my bedroom, where I saw Mom had put a meditation pillow on the floor. It was black and stout in shape, sitting on my rug like a tiny life preserver. I noticed it and promptly ignored it. Call it mother's intuition about what one might face in elementary school, but a few days later I came home crying. Between heaving, dramatic sobs I managed to spit out, "Jessica was so mean to me today. She made fun of my outfit in front of everyone. Why are people so mean? It's not like her clothes are so great! I can never, ever go to school again!" While I can barely remember the details of this incident, I can remember how bad I felt. I was almost inconsolable, the kid version of me believing that a thoughtless and passing comment from a peer would mark me for life as *fashion don't*. I was convinced there was absolutely nothing *anyone in the entire world* could do to make me feel better. My mind was made up; it was impossible for me to go back to school, and my parents would probably need to homeschool me. At that moment, I was drama personified. For my mother, the antidote to these typical elementary school theatrics wasn't a warm hug, words of wisdom, or even a freshly baked cookie, it was meditation. "Emma. Go to your room and meditate for ten minutes. Then we can talk, okay? Remember, just treat your thoughts like clouds passing by. Acknowledge them but don't get too attached to them."

The suggestion that I needed to meditate just fueled my fury. Why couldn't my mother just wrap me in her arms, hug me tight, and let me cry it all out? Or at least let me buy better clothes! But I always did as my mother asked, even if it made me angry. I stomped into my room with my nose running, tears streaming down my bright red face. I plopped my butt down on my meditation cushion with the delicacy of an elephant. Being told to meditate always felt like a double whammy of punishment combined with utter pointlessness. The way I was acting, you would have thought my mother had actually said, "Go to your room, young lady, and don't come out until you've reached enlightenment!" I didn't understand how sitting on this cushion and breathing was going to help me solve my problem with Jessica. I knew my mom wouldn't want to see me for at least ten minutes, so I had to at least go through the motions of meditating. I crossed my legs, sat up straight and tall like my mom did, and just started to breathe through my nose. In and out. In and out. The thoughts that ran through my head were more like bulldogs than fluffy clouds. *School sucks, Jessica is the worst. Why don't I have better pants? Why does Jessica get to be in charge of fashion?* In and out. In and out. *It's just not right to judge someone on the basis of their outfit!* In and out. In and out. *And actually, I don't think there's anything at all wrong with the way I dress.* In and out. In and out. And slowly, the chatter in my mind—about school, meanness, and the arbitrary rules of elementary school fashion—quieted down to the point where I could no longer hear it. My ten-minute, mother-mandated meditation session calmed my breathing and allowed me to sit with my thoughts (even the ugly ones) and breathe through the messy mixture of emotions I was feeling—frustration, anger, sadness, and fear. When I got off my cushion my eyes were still puffy, but the tears had stopped. All of the overwhelming emotions that had caused me so much distress had been knocked down to size. I walked into the kitchen, where my mother was chopping vegetables for dinner. "Oh, how are you feeling, Emma? Want to talk about what happened at school today?" "No. I'm fine. I know what to do. I know how to deal with Jessica. I'm going to start my homework." There was the smallest hint of a smile on Mom's face, like she knew taking ten minutes to meditate had the power to settle the thoughts of the World's Angstiest Kid. The beauty of meditation is self-realization. Especially as a kid who didn't always love advice from my parents, I found that meditation gave me the tools to figure out problems on my own. It can feel overwhelming to think about adding another item into a packed schedule, but I believe there are creative ways to fit meditation seamlessly into your life.

After I had been living in New York City for a few years, one of my friends approached me with an interesting idea.

"Emma, we're going to take a motorcycle riding class in the Bronx so we can get motorcycle licenses! Want to join us?" There were so many physical activities I have tried and enjoyed—snowboarding, paddleboarding, sailing, cycling— but the idea of riding a motorcycle had never crossed my mind. I suddenly pictured myself decked out in leather pants with a matching jacket. I absolutely love learning new things, and I loved the thought of this challenge. It seemed difficult enough, and also thrilling at the same time. I imagined myself a skilled rider, taking huge sweeping turns through large treelined roads in upstate New York, or driving around Soho, stopping at a café, and removing my helmet and setting my hair free. In my mind it was incredibly romantic and badass. Needless to say, I was in for the motorcycle lessons.

My friends and I spent a weekend in the Bronx learning the ins and outs of motorcycle safety. The instructor began the weekend by saying, "If you're good at playing video games you'll probably be good at riding a motorcycle." I didn't grow up with Nintendo in our house but since all of my friends did, I considered myself an expert Mario Cart driver. I thought, *Maybe I'll be good at this?!* The instructor then put the fear of God in each of us, explaining that the stakes are so much higher for motorcycle riders. "There are no airbags, seatbelt, you don't have a roof or bumpers. And unlike a car you've got no crumple zone. A small accident that is no big deal in a car can be a tragedy when you are riding a motorcycle. You have to focus and get good at it if you want to stay alive." I took the idea of learning to ride a motorcycle seriously, but I had to admit that what he said scared me. It sounded like with a single slip of focus, it could all be over. We spent the rest of the weekend learning about basic vehicle function, how to control the motorcycle, how to prepare for different types of weather, and the laws. I immediately saw how different driving a motorcycle really was; you have to be alert and prepared to move very quickly. At the end of the weekend the instructor made a lackluster announcement. "Technically, all of you have passed. But I need to tell you all something. Right now, none of you are great. If you want to get better, you need to practice." After completing the crash course (now there's a horrifying pun) we were all deemed "qualified" to ride a motorcycle, even though our instructor didn't think we were ready to be set loose on the streets of New York City.

The instructor's words kept repeating in my head over and over. How could I practice? Who was going to lend me, a new rider, their motorcycle so I could practice and risk hurting not only myself but their precious motorcycle? I did what any sensible twenty-five-year-old would do and started searching good old Craigslist to see if I could find any motorcycles for sale. This was around the time I had started modeling, so I was actually able to start saving money for this purchase. I can get kind of intense about learning new things, and I knew if I wanted to be great I needed to practice. And if I wanted to practice I needed to buy my own bike. When I told Katie she seemed concerned, but Brad smiled, as if he could picture the two of us flying around town on it together. I found a cute army-green 1979 Honda Twinstar for sale in a beach town on the Jersey Shore. I convinced a friend with a van to drive down with me. When I met the owner and whipped out my checkbook to pay, I quickly learned that Craigslist was more of a cash-only operation. As my friend drove me to ATMs all around town so I could get about $1,400 in cash, I wondered if the universe was saying, *Emma, stop what you're doing. Do not buy a motorcycle!* I pushed the thoughts away, reminding myself that having my own mode of transportation would make life easier, and how fun it would be to be a great and confident rider. A motorcycle would allow me freedom to move through New York City at lightning speed, and that alone would be a win.

The motorcycle instructor's concerns had stayed with me, so I started out cautiously. I slowly rode around some of the quieter, more residential streets of Brooklyn where I felt safer. I even went to the Floyd Bennett airfield in Brooklyn, where I could ride as fast as I wanted with no cars around. Riding a motorcycle is an adjustment; it's almost like driving a stick shift car in the form of an extra heavy and much faster bicycle. I allowed myself to learn slowly and carefully, growing more confident with each ride. I wanted to feel like I was completely in control before I ventured out onto the busier streets. Once I got up the courage to navigate myself into real city traffic, I had to hone my focus down to a molecular level.

I was steering, using a clutch to change gears, and working to maintain my balance while holding my own against
cars, speeding taxis, huge buses, delivery trucks, pedestrians
(many with dogs and/or strollers), and delivery bicycles that
moved at breakneck speed. The traffic pattern was like something out of a video game, except "game over" would mean
I'm dead. Driving a motorcycle in a big city meant processing a million things at once. *Can I legally turn here? Do
cars see me? Can I make this turn without being sideswiped
by a truck? Is that taxi in the next lane going to change
lanes right in front of me?* For a newbie motorcycle rider, it
was overwhelming—there was too much noise, too many
people.

As I stopped at a red light about to head over the Manhattan Bridge into Brooklyn, it started to rain. I realized I was
beginning to panic. Rain and wet roads add a whole other
element to riding that is both uncomfortable and dangerous.
I was worried I wouldn't be in control while riding across the
bridge, and my hands were shaking. As I looked at the cars
around me, and the dry drivers inside of them, I felt like I
could cry. There was just so much going on. I wished I had
windshield wipers and a waterproof jacket! Why did I think
this was a good idea? I forced myself to take a deep breath. I
felt my shoulders relax by just the slightest amount. *Breathe,
Emma. Just breathe. Breathe and focus on the task at hand.*
The light was blissfully long, and I managed to get in a few
rounds of breathing before I had to drive again. I was still

scared, but by remembering to breathe and focus I was able to rein in my fear and regain control. *You know what to do, Emma, you've got this.* During the rest of my journey back to my apartment, I kept breathing and repeating the mantra—just be mindful. I reverted back to the breath, and I stayed alert, focused, calm, and in control. To stay upright and move forward, I had to let that fear and panic go. I made it home soaking wet and unscathed. I parked my motorcycle along the side of my building and realized I felt very calm. The breathing had gotten me through it.

Soon enough I was riding my motorcycle to most of the places I went, meeting Brad for dinner and Katie for yoga, zipping to last-minute auditions, and going back and forth to freelance gigs. I even bought a leather jacket and a pair of brown leather boots with thick sturdy heels. I had a black helmet, and I wore black leather gloves with metal knuckles. I felt powerful, in control, and free. Something I loved about being on that bike was the way I was able to focus and free my mind. It was my urban meditation. When you're riding you can't look at your cell phone or answer a text message. I had no radio; it was just the sound of the wind by my head, and the powerful engine beneath me. I was so aware of my surroundings while also incredibly aware of myself. Sometimes the traffic and driving would give me anxiety, but most of the time it was a perfect way to clear my head and remind myself to just breathe.

As much as I enjoyed it though, my time as that cool girl

who rode a motorcycle was fairly short-lived. While it was convenient in many ways, it was still hard to park it in such a dense urban area, and with traffic, it wasn't always the most practical way to get where I needed to be. I loved that army-green Twin Star, but I went back and forth and back and forth about whether to sell it. While I agonized, the universe decided for me. One day, I came home to my apartment building and discovered it had been stolen. I was sad, but I knew it was probably for the best. And in a moment of grace, I found myself hoping whoever took it would be as careful as I was. And I wished that I could tell whoever was riding it how important it is sometimes to *just breathe*. For years, any time I heard the sound of a motorcycle driving by I would turn my head to look, always hoping I'd see that little green bike once again.

I should probably end on that inspirational note, but I feel I need to add an important coda to my adventures in motorcycle riding. A few years after my bike was stolen, I got a call from my agent to go to a commercial audition for a female who could ride a motorcycle. It was for JCPenney, and I needed to be able to ride with a passenger on the back. I went into that audition pretty confident; there were probably only a handful of women who would be qualified! But unfortunately, I wasn't their first choice (it happens). However, the day before the shoot I received a panicked phone call from the casting director asking if I could come in as a last-minute replacement. It turned out the woman they had hired had *lied* and actually didn't know how to ride a motorcycle. I gladly (and a bit proudly) took the job and got to ride an amazing vintage Triumph motorcycle for a day. Plus there was a cute guy on the back, and the commercial ran nationally for months.

MAKE MINDFULNESS ACCESSIBLE TO YOU

If I could talk to my seven-year-old self who angrily threw her body down on a meditation cushion, I'd tell her that she was learning to use a tool that would be in her arsenal *for life*. Meditation has been my savior at times. It would end up helping me keep anxiety at bay during my mother's cancer treatment. A few rounds of breathing helped me focus and tap into my power before I got started on an eighty-mile fundraising bike ride. And meditation also helped me stay present and enjoy the splendor on my recent trip to Chile. *You are here. Be present and absorb all this beauty around you.* Taking time out of your day to sit and breathe can clear your mind, calm your stress, and help you focus on a difficult task. Meditation is a tool that can support you when you least expect it. If you are in a stressful meeting, remembering to breathe can help you tap into your inner well of confidence and courage. Breathing can center you before a job interview or calm you on a bumpy flight. I have had a regular meditation practice for a long time. I don't get fancy about it (I don't always bother with a cushion!), but I carve time out of my busy life to sit with my breath. Mindfulness can mean something different for everyone, but for me it's about being aware of my emotions, breaking through stress, and being focused on what's in front of me. Think about how full your day is—work, children, family, meetings, deadlines, errands. Life just isn't a stress-free adventure. It comes with tasks, obstacles, and plenty of stress. But if you can learn to have compassion for yourself you can make a difference in your life starting now. You can begin gently. Take a look at your surroundings. What do you see? What do you hear? Remind yourself that this moment is the freest you will ever be. Breathe through it and let your thoughts pass by.

While starting a meditation practice can feel daunting, just remember that there is no goal at the end of it. The only objective is to help you get into a place where you feel peaceful. My experience riding the motorcycle taught me that you don't have to sit on a cushion to focus on the present and let your stress fall away. Performing quiet and soothing activities, or participating in beloved hobbies, can be a great place to start. Get outside and work in the garden. Stick your hands into the dirt, feel its warmth and texture. Let your hands fall into a rhythm as you dig or pull weeds from the earth. If you're a golfer, pay extra attention to your breath as you pull your club back and gracefully swing at that ball. Or focus on the breeze in your hair and the sun on your face as you take a midday walk through your neighborhood. Notice the birds, the plants, and the color of the sky. It doesn't matter how you get to a place of calm. This isn't about having a perfect process, because perfection doesn't exist when it comes to meditation. Meditation isn't about reaching enlightenment either; it's about improving your life today and many tomorrows from now on. Whether you decide to spend ten minutes meditating every day, or you lean into a hobby that sharpens your focus, the benefits will be the same. What matters is that you are giving yourself the opportunity to be mindful. You deserve to be at peace.

A MEDITATION PRIMER, INSPIRED BY EMMA'S MOM, TERESA (NO MOTORCYCLES REQUIRED)

The best part about developing a meditation practice is that it becomes like an old, reliable friend. You might not see each other for a while, but then you meet up and it's just like old times. You fall right into step, you catch up easily, and you leave thinking, *I'm definitely not waiting months to see my BFF Meditation again.* Here is how I was taught to meditate by my mother, and this is how I still practice to this day. I lovingly urge you to try it.

STEP ONE

Find a quiet room and some alone time. I am not kidding at all when I tell you that this is likely the hardest part. Sneak away if you have to, or be on the lookout for little moments that you can carve out of your schedule.

STEP TWO

Sit down on a comfy pillow or chair. If you are on a pillow, sit with your legs crossed. If you're on a chair, sit upright with both feet on the floor. If you can create a regular spot for meditation, that's great. Your meditation space will cue your brain that it's time to relax, but remember that meditation can be done anywhere.

STEP THREE

Lay your left hand on top of your right and let your hands lie in your lap, with your thumbs facing inward. Touch the tips of your thumbs together. This hand position is sometimes called "the cosmic mudra." Your hands should be resting on your lap just below your navel, which is considered the spiritual and energetic center of the body.

STEP FOUR

Close your eyes and breathe normally. Now start to count your breaths, every inhale and exhale counting as one breath. Count to ten breaths, and then start again at number one. The simplicity of this is beautiful, and your practice will only get better over time. Ease into it and enjoy.

A few final words of wisdom from Teresa:

If you'd like, you can visualize the numbers in your head. As you're in the early stages of your meditation practice, this can help to clear your head of other thoughts so you can focus.

Remember! Treat your thoughts like clouds passing by; don't get attached to any one of them.

You must understand that you cannot be "good" at meditating. If your thoughts are wandering and you start thinking of your grocery list, your next meeting, or whether or not your kids are coloring on the wall, that is normal. When you catch your thoughts wandering off, start again at breath number one. No matter how many times it takes, keep coming back to your breath and your counts.

Once you have this down, you can start incorporating different mantras to repeat to yourself over and over again instead of counting.

Remember Emma's advice because it definitely applies here: progress not perfection!

ELEVEN

Don't Sweep Your Feelings Under a Rug

Great music is an essential part of a great workout. I love making playlists for my rides, and I put a lot of thought into it. Creating a playlist with songs I've loved for years and mixing in new artists I'm excited about is one of my favorite parts of my job. But the playlist I was working on for this special ride was different, and the vibe needed to be just right. I was playing "Why" by Annie Lennox, "Breathe Me" by Sia, and "Let It Be" by the Beatles. These songs tugged at my soul and sometimes made me cry, which is exactly what I was going for. Peloton was featuring a series of "mood rides," and I was doing "sad." I thought this ride was important because sadness is an inevitable part of being alive. Sadness hurts, and it's usually a feeling we want to get away from as quickly as we can, but there is value to *feeling* our feelings.

Being human is about experiencing a range of emotions, but I understand how tempting it is to sweep the negative ones under the rug. Why not just stick to the positive ones? Because if you hide feelings away without acknowledging them you just end up with a lumpy rug. When we avoid our feelings, they tend to make their presence known to us by making us anxious, sick, or even depressed. Feelings of sadness, grief, and anxiety are a part of how we process our experiences, and I've worked hard to face these feelings rather than sweep them away. It's never easy, but life is hard enough without having to worry about tripping over a lumpy rug and getting hurt. It's important that we let ourselves feel everything . . . the good and the bad.

Brad and I had been dating for about a year and a half when I noticed his behavior was changing. His jovial, bright personality became muted and dimmed. He was distant and far off. I could feel him pulling away from me, and I didn't know why. I wondered if I had done something wrong, but we hadn't had an argument. Brad had been a guy who always did what he said he was going to do, whether it was call me back or meet me somewhere, but suddenly he wasn't reliable. I found out what was behind this change. After being sober for about two years, Brad had gotten back into drugs. I had no clue how to handle this, but I knew that this was serious. I cared for him so deeply, but it was terrifying and painful to see him falling back into these dangerous habits. It quickly got worse. Brad started disappearing for a few days at a time and wouldn't answer his phone. I would sit in my apartment overwhelmed with anxiety. I didn't know whom he was with, where he was, if he was okay, or even if he was alive. It was an all-encompassing fear. One time, when he'd been gone for four days, I was so worried I asked Katie to walk to his apartment with me. I was practically shaking with fear. "Katie, I have a terrible feeling about this. I don't know what to do." Katie was there for me, assuring me he was probably fine. I still remember how scared I was when we opened the door to his bedroom. I had no idea what we would find. Thankfully, he was okay. He was home, in his dark apartment, but I could tell he was different. After that visit, he called me a few days later. This was the breaking point for me. I couldn't handle the stress. I couldn't handle not knowing where he was and if he was okay. I reached out to his friends and asked for advice, but I felt like there was nothing I could do. I couldn't watch someone I cared about continue to hurt himself. I felt I had no choice; we had to break up. The breakup was hard even though I knew it was the right thing to do at the time. It was painful, but for the sake of my own mental health and my heart, I couldn't remain in that relationship. It was an awful decision to have to make, but I knew it was the right one.

A couple of months later, in August, I got the news I had always hoped would never come. Although Brad and I had broken up, we were still in touch every other day. I was still so worried about him. I hadn't heard from him in two days, and I had the thought, *Maybe he's doing really well. Maybe he's moved on*. It was late morning when one of our mutual friends called me. "Emma, I'm so sorry to tell you this. There is terrible news. Brad overdosed. He's gone. He died." The pain hit me immediately. I hadn't felt this level of emotional distress since the day I came home from school and found the note my dad left on my pillow saying he was leaving us. The grief was overwhelming and it hit me like a crashing wave on shore. When my family of four had been cleaved in two, so had my heart. Now I was once again experiencing an all-encompassing grief that hurt my spirit so much that my body felt all of it. I remember feeling disconnected after that phone call, like it wasn't really happening, even though a part of me always feared this was a possibility. I was home alone, and I completely broke down. I was crying so hard that I struggled to breathe. I threw myself on the couch, amazed by how much it hurt physically. I called Katie and told her what had happened, and she came right home from work to be there with me. I cried nonstop, barely able to believe that someone with Brad's magnetic personality and kindness was gone. My close friends from the island, Nate and Mariah, hopped on a bus from the Cape the first thing the next day. Mariah slept in bed with me for an entire week. I was so distraught that sleeping was nearly impossible, but knowing she was beside me soothed me, and I succumbed eventually. But I'd wake up crying, remembering all over again that Brad's loss was my new reality. I don't know how I would have gotten through that first week without the help of my friends; I don't know how someone could survive that level of pain alone. One evening Katie said to me, "Emma, I know you're hurting so much. I know this is hard to believe in this moment, but this feeling won't last forever. There will be a time that you won't feel this sad." And those words were exactly what I needed to hear. I had been in and out of therapy my whole life. I had spent years talking about the emotional trauma of my parents' divorce, among other things, and I knew what I was experiencing in that moment was profound. I made the decision that I was going to feel these feelings and confront this trauma head on. If I didn't face it now, it might show up five, ten, twenty years from now, and in desperation of feeling completely out of control of my emotions, I made the decision to obsessively take control of my healing.

Katie's words stuck with me. The heaviness of this loss was intense, and it felt like the pain would be with me forever. I couldn't focus; I couldn't work or be present for my friends. I was sitting with all of this sadness, and I could barely manage it. This wasn't something that would just pass; I had to start taking baby steps back into my life. I had to find a way to heal and process what had happened. This wasn't an issue that self-care could conquer, but I thought maybe it could be a starting point. One morning I forced myself to walk to the yoga studio down the block from my apartment. It was the end of summer, and I remember the city felt much quieter than usual, almost like everyone was in mourning with me. I bought a one-month unlimited class package, and I went to yoga every single day that month. For better or for worse, I was going to face this trauma. Sometimes it felt like yoga was making it worse. A simple cat cow exercise or pigeon pose could launch a new set of tears. As we moved through sun salutations, dark thoughts would plague me: *Could I have done something to prevent this? Did I not do enough?* The pain was acute in those moments, but as the days of yoga classes went by, I was able to release some of that guilt and self-blame. I began to think about the good moments. Toward the end of the month, I started to experience some happy memories of Brad too. In resting poses, I could see his smile. I deeply missed the carefree guy that I had loved, who would stay up goofing off and dancing the night away with me. Sometimes these memories made me cry more; other times I felt myself smile. Brad was a special person, who loved deeply, who *felt* deeply, but he suffered from a sickness. His addiction took over his life, and so much of his time, energy, and personality became consumed by his drug habit. There was nothing I could have done, but knowing this didn't make the pain disappear. In addition to the yoga, I took other positive actions to support myself while I was processing this grief. I went to therapy twice a week, and I wrote down all of my feelings.

DON'T SWEEP FEELINGS UNDER THE RUG, YOU'LL JUST END UP WITH A LUMPY RUG

Yoga alone does not cure grief. No one thing can, but that doesn't mean we will stay mired in grief when the unthinkable happens. Living a full life means being subjected to disappointments, frustrations, and heartbreak, as well as moments of joy and excitement. It's so tempting to numb ourselves during difficult times, with alcohol, food, or even flat-out denial. When Brad died, I didn't want to feel deeply because it hurt too much. But it hurt that much because I had *cared so deeply*. It often doesn't seem like it, but our ability to feel deeply as human beings is a gift—even the emotions that are almost impossible to tolerate. Sweeping them away has the potential to cause more harm, because you're not getting rid of them, you're letting them simmer inside of you. Things that continue to simmer have the potential to boil over and leave you with a big mess. It is easy to believe that happiness is always supposed to be the leader of our emotions. Happiness is a wonderful and important part of what it means to be human, but it's not the full picture. To be human is to experience a huge range of emotions, and no feelings are wrong. Whatever you are experiencing is valid. But when you find yourself in that dark place where grief, sadness, anxiety, and disappointment live, remember this isn't where you are going to stay. Remember that this is one moment. Take a step toward healing yourself. Get help, ask for support, cry, honor your memories, reflect, and take inventory of your own life. While there is no timeline for emotions to shift, know that with self-kindness and support, you will eventually find yourself at peace.

Fatefully, as I was reflecting on what I wanted to say about this time in my life, my sister-in-law, Jenn (who somehow knew I needed inspiration before I knew it), forwarded me a quote from James Clear's weekly newsletter that really stood out to me: "The brilliance of the stars would be invisible without the vast darkness of space behind them. Do not wish away the difficult portions of life. They provide the contrast needed to appreciate the joyful moments."

Brad's death changed my life, but eventually grief loosened its grip on me. I will never forget him or the joy he brought to my life. Knowing Brad showed me how deeply I can feel, and I'm grateful for that. When I led that Sad Ride, the loss I was talking about was Brad's death. After that ride so many people shared their feelings and I was glad to know that my experience with grief could help others. One woman reached out about the pain of losing her husband suddenly in her early thirties. Another man shared that he had lost his wife to cancer and told me about his two beautiful children and how they were picking up the pieces together. I was grateful to have an outlet to share my story, and I appreciate everyone who listened and cried with me over those gut-wrenching songs during that ride.

Music can so often unlock feelings we didn't know we had, and as gut-punching as it can be when we're feeling sadness and pain, it can also be the art form that intrinsically captures our joys and our loves. One of my favorite things about

Dave is that he is just as passionate about music as I am. He plays the guitar casually and gets just as excited as I do about seeing our favorite bands in concert. He played Division I football in college and knows something about songs that get people pumped up. He's my go-to resource when I need a song that will keep riders motivated, whether it's AC/DC or the Red Hot Chili Peppers. But our mutual love of music goes beyond Dave's helping me with playlists. We've taken countless road trips together listening to our favorite nineties playlist. We're both big Foo Fighters fans, and they are often heavily featured on those playlists. Since I met Dave, the song "Everlong" has evolved from *just a song I love* to a song that brings back instant memories of our relationship as it's grown from something brand-new to a truly loving partnership. The opening chords of that song conjure up memories of cruising up to Rhode Island or spending hours together building our new kitchen. There are countless songs we love—I could never narrow it down to just one—but knowing that Dave Grohl wrote the song about "being connected to someone so much, that . . . when you sing along with them you harmonize perfectly" makes it even more meaningful. That song lifts my heart, and I believe it will always be a part of the soundtrack of the life we continue to build together.

TWELVE

Home Is in Your Heart

It was early in the evening on Martha's Vineyard and I was on one of my semiregular summer visits, sitting on my mom's porch listening to the soundtrack of my life—the robins, chickadees, and cardinals singing . . . accompanied by the *whoosh-whoosh* of the sprinkler. I was perched on one of the old wicker chairs with its faded blue cushion when I caught a big whiff of privet hedges mixed with wild honeysuckle that immediately made me feel at home. The porch plants were bursting with life and the grapevines hung gracefully off the side of the porch, creating a secret haven for sitting. Above my head hung Mom's wicker basket collection, and on my lap was a bowl of her lo mein. The combination of noodles, shredded veggies, chicken, sesame oil, and soy sauce was perfection. I had just stuck my chopsticks into my noodles when I heard the ping of a text message. It was my dad. "Emma, can't wait to see you. Fishing this weekend?" I responded with a yes, even though I knew it meant an early wake-up, just as I got another message from an old friend. "What time do you want to meet for dinner tonight?" I took another bite of noodles, and I heard my mother puttering around in her kitchen. I thought, *It feels so good to be back home,* surrounded by people whom I have loved for years.

"Home" can be a tricky concept, even though it shouldn't be. For a long time, I struggled to understand where home really was for me. On the Vineyard I was Emma Lovewell aka Teresa and Mark's kid, Alan's sister, the lifeguard, bartender, and lip-synching champion. I stayed with my mother whenever I visited the island, and while I always felt comfortable in the home where I grew up, sometimes I remembered that the happy family of four who lived under this roof didn't exist anymore. There were happy memories in that house, but some dark ones too. In New York City I was one of millions trying to make her way, build a career, and figure out who she was. My home in New York had been a series of different small apartments shared with different people. I never stayed in any of them long enough to create a space that really reflected who I was. Everything was temporary. Then one summer, a few years ago, I unexpectedly found myself living on the Vineyard for several months, when my mom was sick. Her illness was one of the toughest experiences my family has gone through, but I learned a crucial lesson about what home really means. Many of us struggle to find a place where we truly belong, but it's not about where you sleep or keep your stuff. To feel truly at home in the world, you need to embrace and cherish the times when your heart felt the fullest.

One of the apartments in New York that proved to be unexpectedly temporary was the first one Dave and I moved into together many years ago. It was exciting to be building a shared space, settling into new routines, and creating little rituals of our own. Tompkins Square Bagels was a few blocks away and we often stopped by to grab one of the most delicious New York City bagels before heading to Tompkins Square Park to find a bench to eat. This bagel shop always had the freshest bagels, so they refused to toast them for you because they were already warm from the oven. There was always this interesting dynamic in the park, watching the squirrels and then the rats run by. I always wondered if they were in competition, were friends, or just tolerated each other. Overhead a red-tailed hawk would fly by, and Dave and I would narrate this wild but urban scene as if we were David Attenborough on *Planet Earth*. We each liked the city as much as we liked the outdoors. We loved taking advantage of the art, culture, food, and music in New York, but were equally delighted to surf and swim on summer trips to the beach. We were happy about the life we were creating together, but we were a little stuck in the career department. Neither of us was sure about how to get to the next level. We were both passionate about fitness and start-ups, and we were ready for a new adventure. I had been teaching cycling classes almost nonstop for years, but I thought there had to be something bigger for me out there. Dave was working in operations at the same fitness company and was ready to look for something new and was curious to explore unknown horizons. We had a few opportunities arise, even internationally, and when something interesting for both of us popped up in Texas, we were intrigued but highly cautious as well. We had never considered moving to Texas before, but we were ready for a change and thought this could be a temporary move for us—make some sacrifices, learn some new skills, save some money, and then move on to another project. The job was to help build a new fitness studio for expansion. The challenge of starting something new out of the city appealed to both of us, and we planned to take hiking trips in places we'd always wanted to spend more time—like New Mexico and Colorado. It would be a major change of scenery in all ways, but we were excited for a fresh start.

We were finalizing our road-trip plans when the phone rang. I knew something was wrong the second I heard my godmother, Dianne's, voice. "Emma, it's Dianne. I think you should come home now. Your mom just went to the hospital. She's not doing well. Her nose is bleeding, and it won't stop." My stomach dropped. I had a bad feeling about this. I stopped packing and checked the ferry schedules. If I hurried, Dave and I could drive to the Cape in time for the last ferry. When I got to the island my mom was in the emergency room, and it was around ten P.M. They had put cotton gauze, basically a tampon, in her nose to try to stop the bleeding, but it wasn't working. I lay next to her in her hospital bed, held her hand, and put some classical music on my phone, which always seemed to soothe her. I didn't know if I said the right thing, but I knew we were both scared. My mom looked small and tired, and with worry in her voice she said, "Emma, they think this might be related to allergies." After I brought her home I got her settled in bed and immediately called my brother. We agreed that we couldn't assume this was related to allergies and that we needed to get Mom to the mainland to see a specialist right away. I started calling people we knew on the island to see if anyone could recommend someone. Each time I heard a familiar voice on the phone I felt a little bit of comfort; there were so many people on the island who loved and cared about my mother—but no one had any answers. Finally, I called the ear, nose, and throat department of Mass General Hospital in Boston. They were able to get me an emergency appointment the next day. Living on an island is always challenging, and because we didn't have a ferry reservation we woke up extra early to wait on standby in hopes we could get off the island to head to Boston. Thankfully we were able to get her to the hospital the next day, and the specialist was able to tell us that, unfortunately, my mother had a tumor in her sinuses. After multiple exams, tests, and surgery, and weeks of me traveling back and forth from New York to the island, my mom was diagnosed with an aggressive form of cancer.

When the call came that the tumor was cancerous, I felt like I had been punched in the gut. I was so scared, but I decided I would do whatever it took to get my mom safely through this crisis. My brother flew in from California and my dad came over too. The four of us stood in the living room crying in a big group hug. My parents had been divorced for years, but all of us standing together reminded me of how much love we still shared. It was hard to believe that this was the same room where we celebrated Chinese New Year and listened to my dad playing guitar when we were kids. Now we were reunited because my mother was seriously ill. There were lots of plans to make. Mom's treatment would require radiation and another surgery, which meant frequent trips to the mainland. Mom also had her own gardening business, and it needed to stay afloat during her treatment so she wouldn't lose her source of income.

This wasn't what I had anticipated, but I had no doubt about what I needed to do, and Dave was completely on board. We adjusted our plan. I would move home and take over my mother's gardening business so my mom could stay in Boston at my aunt's house to receive treatment five days a week. During this time, Dave would go to Texas to work and get our stuff in order, and I'd join him in September. I spent the following months driving around the island in my mom's pickup truck, planting annuals, watering garden beds, pruning and weeding, trimming shrubs, and tending to the delicate needs of temperamental roses. I'd often be kneeling in the dirt when a client would walk into the backyard. "Emma, how is your mother? We are all thinking of her." Every person I talked to on the island adored my mother and was keeping us all in mind. As I deadheaded annuals, I thought about the childhood moments I had spent gardening with my mother, seething with resentment. How perfect that all of that hard work Mom made me do had put me in a position to be able to protect her livelihood when she needed help. As I snipped away, I wondered, *What* will *my livelihood be? Will I ever feel rooted to one place and one profession?* I had such high hopes for our new situation in Texas. Maybe I'd no longer be floating along, and I could finally stop worrying about what came next.

After a long day of gardening in the sun, I'd drive my mother's truck to the dump to toss all of the clippings, grass, and branches, then I would head back home. Inevitably there would be something waiting for me on the porch, a bag of veggies from a neighbor's garden or a loaf of homemade bread with a note, *We are all thinking of you. Let us know if you need anything at all.* Even though I was exhausted and desperate for a shower, these gestures always perked me up and made me smile. My friends who live on the island checked on me constantly, inviting me over for cookouts or get-togethers on the beach. They knew I was living in my child-hood home alone and what I really needed was my community. Dad called daily to see how things were going. My brother too. My mom would check in every day to tell me about treatment and to ask me about every single client's garden. Everywhere I turned there was someone who cared about me and my family. I thought about the home I had built in New York. I remember walking down the street soon after I first moved there, amazed by the number of people on the streets, jogging, eating brunch, walking dogs, or having drinks with friends. There was so much *living* happening all around me, but I still felt like an outsider. I knew a handful of people, but it could be lonely. It was a long time before I met Katie, who became someone I could lean on as I navigated my new life. I lived with Katie for five years. She could finish my sentences and had been there for some of the best and worst moments of my life. Now I was moving away from her. What would it be like moving to a place where I didn't know anyone? I wasn't just leaving a city, I was leaving the people who knew me best, and that was terrifying.

HOME *IS* SOMETHING YOU CAN TAKE WITH YOU

A few weeks later, after I'd scrubbed the dirt off myself in the shower and fixed myself something to eat, I started tidying the house because Mom would be coming home tomorrow and staying until her next treatment. Mom got to come home between treatments thanks to the pilots from Angel Flight, who took my mother back and forth from the island on the weekends. We thanked them with homemade jam because there were no words to describe how grateful we were for their help. As I was dusting the bookshelf in my bedroom, I noticed something that looked familiar. As I reached for a book with a faded yellow spine and pulled it out, I knew exactly what it was. It was my journal from when I was ten years old. I sat down on my bed and opened it to a page that read,

> Today I practiced piano for 30 minutes. Then I listened to my Alanis cassette. Alan was playing computer. Mom made pasta for dinner while dad was playing guitar. Alan and I fought over the last shrimp. At dinner dad told a bad joke but we laughed anyway.

I flipped through the worn pages, barely able to recognize my childhood scrawl. I fought back a tear as I realized I was holding my life story in my hands. My ten-year-old self wrote down her memories, her fears, her hopes, and the day-to-day minutiae that add up to a life. The small, everyday moments I had written about transported me right back to childhood. I could practically smell my mother's pasta sauce simmering and hear the sound of Alanis Morissette's voice from my cassette player. I took a moment to reflect on how I was wrapping up a big stage in my life just as another was about to begin. My time on the Vineyard was nearing an end. Mom's treatment was almost over, and it was just about time to meet Dave in Texas. I didn't know what to expect there, but I knew I was ready to tackle whatever it was with Dave at my side. That journal was a reminder that stories, like life, take unexpected turns . . . illnesses, divorces, job changes, big moves. These foundational moments are important and sometimes life altering. But the big events don't make up your entire narrative. It's the day-to-day, uneventful moments that are the true building blocks of our stories. It's the *living* that adds the true flavor, zest, and richness to life . . . the long walks, the late-night conversations, the shared meals. The beautiful collection of memories that have been imprinted on my heart is like carrying "home" with me wherever I go. My memory of fighting over the last shrimp with my brother means more than any of the books on my shelves or the clothes in my closet. The post-dinner ice cream runs with Dave are more meaningful to me than anything we've bought for our new house. Memories of sailing with Dad and gardening with Mom are more important than any gift they could give me. These scenes from my life story keep me anchored to the world no matter where I am.

I've always kept a journal, and I like to take a few minutes each morning to write about what I'm grateful for. It's a habit that has made me a more positive and appreciative person. Now I see this small practice as something much bigger. Journaling is a reminder that our life stories can change every single day. We can't control the unexpected events life tosses at us, but we can be deliberate about the rest of our stories. We have the power to craft a life story that reflects our values, passions, and purpose. We have the ability to reflect on our stories and think, *Is this the narrative I really want to follow? Is this the story I want?* I was nervous about the big, new chapter Dave and I were embarking on and about leaving the city behind. Whatever this new chapter threw at us, we didn't have to let it define our entire story. The little details were up to us, and I knew those were the ones that mattered most. Whatever happened in our next chapter, it was a part of the life we were building *together*. The memories of our experience, both good and bad, would become part of *our* story.

STOCK YOUR ASIAN PANTRY: A PRIMER

I grew up watching my mom teach other people to cook Chinese food in our kitchen on Martha's Vineyard. When I was a kid, there weren't many options for Asian food, so Mom decided to change that by showing people how to cook some of her favorite dishes, like dumplings, lo mein, and kung pao chicken. I used to marvel at how Mom could transform the same basic ingredients into so many kinds of dishes. Having these ingredients in my home always makes it feel more like, well, home. This is why I always make sure my pantry is stocked with the following:

Soy sauce

Shaoxing wine (rice wine)

Black rice vinegar

Hoisin sauce

Fermented bean paste

Oyster sauce

Dried chilis

Dried mushrooms

Fish sauce

Star anise

Chili bean paste

Cellophane noodles

Egg noodles

Dumpling wrappers

Rice

Scallions

Garlic

Fresh ginger

Sesame oil

THIRTEEN

Write Your Goals in Pencil

My schedule had been packed all summer with running my mom's gardening business and helping usher her through treatment. The treatment was considered successful, but they were still talking about a round of chemotherapy, just to be safe. Luckily the hospital on the island would be able to administer it, so my mom would be able to get treatment locally. Now that Mom was back home, I realized how sluggish I felt. My energy was depleted. I forced myself out of bed and made a cup of coffee to take out to the porch to drink in the cool morning air. I was well aware of what my problem was, and I didn't want to face it. I hadn't exercised for a few days, and it was taking a toll on me. The sun was shining and there was a good breeze. I wanted to be outside and enjoy the weather, so I told myself that after that cup of coffee I was putting on my shoes and taking a run. Here is my deep, dark secret. I don't enjoy running and I envy people who do enjoy it. The simplicity of exercising outside and needing nothing but shoes is appealing, but I've never taken to it. Now, running after a ball is different. I "get" running as part of a game. But long-distance running has never come easily to me. Nevertheless, sometimes it's the most readily available form of exercise, and at that moment I just needed to get moving.

I started jogging down Mom's driveway toward a pretty road that doesn't see too much traffic. There was a five-mile out and back that I'd walked that would be long enough to get really breathless and recenter myself. After I felt my legs loosen up, I quickened my pace. I felt like I'd been running forever, but it'd only been a few minutes. I told myself to *just do it and move,* and I focused on putting one foot in front of the other. I kept going, trying to enjoy the scenery and the weather, but making it to the halfway point felt impossible. I let myself slow down a bit, but I kept running. I hit the half-way mark, but I couldn't believe it had taken me as long as it did. I had to face the fact that I was miserable, and I decided to walk home. I was frustrated and annoyed with myself. *What is wrong with me? I can do cardio on the bike! I am a fitness professional! People count on me to help them reach their goals and I can't even finish a run?*

When I finally got home after what felt like an epic jour-ney, I found my mom sitting on the porch. "Oh, you're back!

You were gone longer than I thought." I felt like every drop of sweat that was pouring out of me smelled like failure. "Yeah. Well, I had to walk most of the way and it was five miles." Mom took a sip from her mug of tea. "Oh, well, that's great that you got five miles in. Well done. Are you going to take a shower?" I stretched out in the yard, even though I'd barely run, and headed inside to grab a towel. I took a long outdoor shower underneath the grapevines overhead, letting the sweat and the frustration wash away. I thought about what Mom said and I started to feel better. It might not have been my best workout, but I did move and sweat. I just walked more than I ran. I didn't crush my goal of running five miles, but it didn't mean I'd failed. I just needed to adjust my goals (at least for now). I could always do another workout tomorrow.

As a fitness coach it is my job to push you, and I want to be the first in line to congratulate you when you nail a goal, beat your personal record, or have a milestone ride. It's important to have high expectations for yourself, but there are times when we need to accept and appreciate what's currently available to us. As someone who has been known to stumble home from a run, I know that there are instances when our goals need to be flexible. Sometimes we need to give ourselves that extra push, and other times goals need to be adapted to our circumstances. I learned this on a small scale during that Vineyard run and on a very large scale in Texas, when our experience there completely altered the approach I take to setting goals, with fitness as well as the rest of my life. I discovered it's a great service to myself to write my goals in pencil. Literally and metaphorically. To write them, yes, and speak them, and pursue them, but know that sometimes they can change, and that is okay.

With my mother's health crisis safely behind us for now (she was cancer-free after completing two rounds of treatment), I was off to the Lone Star State to reunite with Dave and jump right into our new project. Landing in Texas was a little shocking. The heat felt so intense, and the flat, expansive land was the opposite of the dewy, green landscape of Martha's Vineyard, where I had spent the summer. "Wait until you see our house!" Dave and I had picked out this cute rental at the end of a cul-de-sac, but I hadn't seen it since he moved all of our stuff in. When Dave pulled into the driveway, I couldn't believe the house in front of me was ours. Our rental house had three bedrooms, two baths, a large kitchen, a two-car garage, and, almost unbelievably to me . . . a swimming pool. And yes, it was still far cheaper than any of our New York City one-bedroom apartments. I was exhausted from my travels and frazzled from the change, and I knew a solid workout would put me in a better state of mind. I did a quick Google search and found a fitness studio nearby. I grabbed a sports bra, T-shirt, and leggings from my suitcase, and Dave and I headed to this fitness studio in a neighborhood we had never been in before. I was hoping that some movement would make me feel like my regular self soon enough. Dave and I were both on our treadmills. I was walking first and then transitioned into a quick jog. I worked up a serious sweat, so I took off my T-shirt. I fell into a rhythm and decided I was properly warmed up and could start the rest of the circuit. I started to slow down, and I felt a presence standing next to me. I glanced to the side and saw the instructor, a woman with large muscles and a name tag. I slowed down to a walk and made eye contact with her. "Ma'am, you'll need to put your top back on immediately. This is a family-friendly establishment." I felt embarrassment rush over me and quickly spat out an "Oh! Um, of course! I didn't know!" I put my shirt back on over my very sweaty body. I felt people looking at me, and I couldn't shake the feeling that I was being judged. I reminded myself I came to the gym to work out, to feel better, and I tried to get myself back in the zone. I decided to stay on the treadmill to try and shake off this bad feeling. I started to jog again, ignoring the eyes I still felt on me. A poster on the other side of the gym caught my eye. I looked around and realized that there were posters all over the gym featuring provocative photos of women working out in revealing gym clothes. I looked at what I was wearing. My sports bra fell squarely into crop top territory, and it was high neck as well, hiding all of the necklaces I was wearing. All that was showing of my body was my belly button. My embarrassment started to turn into anger. Was there something about *my* specific belly button that made it not family-friendly? Was "family-friendly" a way of saying, "We don't want you here if you're different"? Was she trying to make me feel insecure about my body? I stopped the treadmill, feeling too angry to stay put. As a fitness instructor myself, I took pride in creating safe workout environments where people of all shapes and sizes are welcome and feel comfortable. I couldn't believe how out-of-place this woman had just made me feel in her studio and in my own body. I had just wanted to make myself feel better about the crazy change happening in my life, but instead I'd been shamed about my body. I walked out of that gym, and I knew I would never go back.

One of the greatest gifts my mother has given me is a positive body image. Growing up near beaches, I was used to running around in a swimsuit and thinking nothing of it. My mom always sat on the beach proudly and without self-consciousness. For Mom, going to the beach was about taking her kids to swim, being active, and having fun. If she had neglected to shave her legs or armpits she didn't care. My mom was unapologetic and carefree with herself in a way that empowered me to be comfortable with my own body. My mother never criticized her own body either, and I am grateful for this. Shame around our bodies is contagious and unhealthy. In high school, it was common that girls would criticize their appearances. One girl would say, "I hate my eyes," and then another would say, "I hate my thighs." When

I was asked, "Emma, what do you hate about your body?" I felt confused, because I didn't spend much time or energy hating on myself. I only became negatively aware of my body when other people would comment on it. We are often taught to think badly about our bodies far before we are taught to love our bodies. When I studied abroad in China, I gained a few pounds because of my change in diet and lifestyle. I knew I had gained weight, but I wasn't that worried about it. I went to see a guy I had been dating after I landed back in the States, and I'll never forget the look on his face when he saw me. "Oh, wow. So, I guess you gained some weight while you were away? Are you going to go on a diet?" No, I wasn't going to go on a diet (though I was definitely going to lose him!). Life is too short to be hungry. I was going to be kind to myself by eating nutritious, delicious foods and exercising like I always had. There was no room in my life for someone who couldn't handle my shifting body.

LOVE YOURSELF INTO CHANGE, WRITE YOUR GOALS IN PENCIL

One of the biggest compliments I have ever received came from a belly-button-baring woman who took one of my cycling classes. She walked up to me after class one day and I recognized her from taking my classes every week. She said, "I'm so comfortable in your class. I'm a size eighteen and I never imagined I'd feel free enough to work out in just a sports bra—but I do in your class. I love my body for what it can do! Thank you, thank you!"

Those words made my heart sing, because that is what fitness is about: being good to yourself, respecting your body, and taking care of it. You cannot hate yourself into change, you'll only end up burying yourself in shame. If you want to change your fitness levels or grow leaner or stronger, you've got to *love yourself* to get to your goal. If you're having trouble meeting a goal, whether it's to increase muscle mass or train for a marathon, be kind to yourself and change your plan, or even change your goal! Write your goals in pencil. Give yourself more time. Only you get to decide what your goals look like. Your body is what carries you through this world, and while I want to help you stay strong and healthy— never forget to love yourself the way you are right now.

And when you alter your goals, sometimes a big dose of self-love is what will get you over that finish line. It surprised me how quickly I was able to feel shame for having a belly button *like everyone else on the entire planet*. I bounced back quickly because I know my body is something to be proud of, if for no other reason than the simple fact that it's mine.

I arrived home from the gym determined to put the incident behind me and focus on what we were there to do. But just a few days after my arrival it became blaringly apparent that this new venture was not the right one. I thought we would be focusing on expansion, and it turned out the whole company was imploding and hanging on by a thread.

I looked around our new house. All of my things were still packed up in boxes—my clothes, dishes, pots and pans, books, and every random object I've collected in my life. Dave and I looked at each other, realizing we needed a new plan. "Emma, this is why we write our goals in pencil," Dave said. "It wasn't meant to be and we can change course. We've always wanted to try out California, what do you say?"

We hadn't failed, we just needed to alter our plans. As you know already, our dreams for California *also* didn't pan out. Another opportunity that wasn't quite what we thought it would be. Regroup. Erase. Try again. "Hey, why don't you email Peloton?" Fresh sheet of paper. New pencil. New plan. We headed back to New York, "Peloton instructor" written in pencil. I hoped it would finally be the dream I could trace over in ink.

FOURTEEN

Have More Best Days

Dave and I were finally settling into our new home. We had spent hours renovating our kitchen, painting walls, creating a small studio where I could make video content, and planting my dream garden. My mother's seventieth birthday was coming up, and since the house was ready, I wanted to throw her a big party. I wrote out a guest list and booked a caterer. Dave and I worked nonstop hanging lights and decorations so that our backyard looked like something out of a romantic comedy. The sun was in the western sky as the first guests arrived, and the twinkling lights looked magical against the pale-purple sky. The table on our deck was covered with a feast: some of my mom's favorite Taiwanese dishes, lots of colorful salads, big wedges of cheese, oysters, dumplings, and the birthday party requisite noodles, which represent living a long life. My mom was happily chatting with her guests, and I smiled because in a few minutes there was going to be a big surprise. The day before, we'd decided to hire a mariachi band. I saw Dave wave to me from inside of the house. "Emma, the band just got here!" He joined me on the porch and put his arm around me; we couldn't wait to see the look on my mother's face. The mariachi band emerged from behind the house in their black and red suits with gold trim and big hats. It was quite an entrance, and their outfits alone added to the festive vibe. Mom started dancing to "Las Mañanitas," and everyone looked over and started to laugh and clap. My mother's face lit up with the surprise and she was glowing. So jubilant, so full of health. The band transitioned into "La Bamba," and I watched my mother dance freely, surrounded by all the people she loved most. My brother and his wife, her grandson, Dave's family, my grandmother Po Po and several of her siblings. Not only was my mother the center of attention, but she was proudly showing off her family too. Mom was introducing us to anyone we didn't know well and sharing a laundry list of accomplishments. "Did you know that Alan is the CEO of his very own company? And Emma has found such success! Her career is taking off! Have you met my grandson, Luca? He's over there with his mom. He's such a smart little boy, and you must meet my lovely daughter-in-law!"

My mother moved around freely to the music, her happiness splashed across her face and her joy infectious. She'd taught me so much, and now as I watched her glide across the lawn, I wondered if my love for music and dance came from her too. Mom has taken ballroom dance lessons on the Vineyard on and off for years. She can fox-trot, box step, and waltz, and she loves to tell me which dance goes with which song. Just as my mom and I were beginning to waltz together, the band leader shouted, "Are there any requests out there?" My mom responded by shouting back, "Yes, please play 'Feliz Navidad'!" Christmas was still months away, but somehow it seemed appropriate that everyone was laughing and singing "I want to wish you a Merry Christmas" as we celebrated my mother's seventieth birthday on a warm September night.

The dancing, drinking, eating, and fun continued. My entire yard filled with the sounds of people celebrating *my mother,* and my heart swelled with gratitude. Finally, after that light-purple sky had turned to black, there was a birthday cake, singing, and candles. As my mom took a deep breath to blow out her candles, I wondered what she'd wished for. I hoped she got it. After the cake was served, the makeshift dance floor of newly laid sod started to empty out. One by one people hugged and kissed my mother goodbye; the long line of people waiting to express their love for her was a beautiful sight. Finally, the last hug was given, and Mom's celebration came to a close. The night was flawless. I walked over to my mother and said, "Happy birthday. I love you, Mom." She looked back at me and said, "Emma, I think this was the best day of my life." I felt a tear threaten to drop down my face. "Mom, I am so glad! It was great." We walked inside together, and I couldn't help but think, *My mother deserves to have more Best Days.* We all deserve more best days. Not every day can be about parties and presents, and it's not every day that we crush a major goal or hit some sort of big milestone. But after my mother's birthday party I was determined to have a Best Day more frequently. I didn't want to limit myself to an occasional "best day of my life." I wanted to celebrate joy on a daily basis without the need for a huge life event. I have learned many lessons from my mother, but I am grateful that her joy that night made me think about how to embrace and enjoy the big moments and the small ones.

I stood on the sidewalk outside of the Peloton studio weighing my options. I had some time before I needed to head home to have dinner with Dave, and I decided to make the most of it. I tossed around the idea of visiting a museum or shopping, but then I remembered there was a dance studio nearby that I'd wanted to check out. I looked at their schedule, and when I saw there was a class starting in fifteen minutes, I decided it must be *fitness fate* and I headed over. It was a Monday afternoon, but the studio had the amped-up energy of a Friday night dance party. I took a spot in the back, and a smile spread across my face as I registered everyone around me. There were people of all shapes, sizes, and colors. Some people, like me, were wearing basic shorts or sweats and T-shirts; other people were so decked out they looked like they were going to a rave. I saw some flashy gold lamé, some leopard print, and even 1980s-style neon tights with high-cut leotards.

The music started and we all followed along with the instructor. There was an instant charge in the air as people start wooing and clapping. Once we'd repeated some of the moves a few times, people started to add their own flair. There was plenty of hip swinging, booty shaking, and twerking. Something happens when you move your body to music, whether you're bopping around your living room alone or have a total stranger twerking-for-the-sake-of-their-life right next to you. The music was clearing my head while simultaneously pumping me up and relaxing me. Moving your body to music *is magical*. The positive energy spread around the class as we all sweated and moved together. I was having such a great time, my mood was so good that I felt like I could do anything. After forty-five heart-pumping minutes, we hit the cool down, and I was high from dancing.

I was still buzzing from all the good energy when I walked out of the studio, all aglow from my sweat and the music. I was instantly thrown back into the thick of life; the streets were packed with people, and I was energized by *all of the living* going on around me. I popped into a very cute coffee shop. As I waited in line for my matcha latte, I heard the constant clacking of keyboards, like every table housed a mini start-up. I imagined what everyone was doing while they were sipping on art-foam-topped cappuccinos. Writing a business proposal, planning a retreat, writing a love letter or maybe a novel? I heard my name and moved forward to get my latte. I took a sip and walked down the street enjoying the pulse of the city, but then it was time to head home.

I listened to my calming playlist as I headed out of the city just past rush hour. What was left of the sun glowed in the sky to my west. As I got closer to home, the sides of the road became lusher and greener, and the sky felt higher without all the skyscrapers taking up all the space. I pulled into the driveway at dusk. I saw a glow from the lights in the kitchen. Dave was probably making dinner. I walked in the front door and Kimchi and Rhody, my new kitty, were the first to greet me. "Hi, you're home. Your brother sent fish! It will be ready in ten. Just relax and then we can eat." We are often the lucky recipients of Alan's generosity from his sustainable seafood company, Real Good Fish. I sat at the kitchen counter and Rhody leapt onto my lap, purring. I took a deep breath and inhaled the smell of olive oil and garlic and roasting vegetables. The intensity of the city had slipped away, the sounds of traffic replaced by the calming sound of Dave's knife chopping vegetables on the cutting board. Dave served me baked fish with sweet potatoes and broccoli. My plate was full of color and tasted like contentment. We sat together at the island we'd installed with our own hands, and I couldn't help but marvel at this life that we had built together. Between bites, Dave asked, "How was your day?" I sat back and told him about the dance class and the live ride I had done earlier in the day. "I haven't done a dance class like that in so long. It was fun! My live ride today went really well too. By the way, I found a new coffee shop. They have mushroom coffee! But I stuck with matcha." I looked at Kimchi and Rhody curled up together on the couch and noticed the moonlight shining through the patio door. "This dinner is great. Thank you for making it. I think this is the perfect ending to what has been a Best Day." Dave smiled. "Can I eat the rest of the fish?" We turned the conversation to Dave's day, then discussed what we wanted to do for the upcoming weekend and talked about renovating the laundry room. I cleared the table and loaded the dishwasher, thinking, *Maybe I'll have a Best Day this weekend too.*

Not every day is for breaking records, not every day will be *the* Best Day, but if you adjust your mindset even slightly, you will have more Best Days. When you think about it, the idea that something should be "the best day of your life" is filled with pressure. Weddings, graduations, births of children—so many expectations, and what if they aren't met? Why do we put so much pressure on ourselves to have unmatchable, Best anythings? If you can adjust to the idea of having a Best Day, you can be open to finding little joys and delights. If any day can be a Best Day, then it takes the focus off of everything having to seem so momentous and consequential. A Best Day is something you can celebrate all the time, and I want you to have more of them. Don't let a bummer of a workout derail you from seeing the value of it. Don't let an imperfection sour your day when everything else is full of sweetness and light. Just keep riding, keep trying, and when all else fails—make a cup of tea and just sit down and have a chat with someone you love. It doesn't get much better than that.

FIFTEEN

Love Yourself, Treat Yourself, Date Yourself

A visit to my acupuncturist always goes the exact same way. He examines my palms and then asks me to stick out my tongue. "You're running hot, Emma. All New Yorkers run hot!" He asks me to lie back as he gets ready to insert needles into different acupuncture points on my body. They are gently tapped into my feet, forehead, and legs—I barely feel them go in. I close my eyes and relax, thinking peaceful thoughts about the energy that is moving around in my body. While I don't quite drift off, I feel a lightness inside of me—almost like I've been mentally and physically decluttered. *Less hot*. It's very rare for any of us to carve time out of our day to really digest things—to take note of the emotions we've felt and experiences we've had. We operate on a high level constantly, everything happening so fast we can't take stock of what we're letting in. And our brains and bodies are always working! There are so many things to think about and so many responsibilities to handle that we don't pay attention to the energy that is constantly coursing through our systems. I like to think of energy as a life force that you can plug into and be revitalized by, but it's also true that if you never disconnect you can feel depleted. Everything must be able to flow back and forth. Unwinding is becoming increasingly difficult to do, as modern life is a never-ending series of distractions and duties. To keep balanced we all need to take care of ourselves, we all need to pay attention to the needs of the body, mind, and spirit. But to stay healthy and happy we all need to do something bigger. I am happier and healthier when I take the time to love myself, treat myself, and even date myself (I'll explain what that means soon).

LOVE YOURSELF

The act of self-love is powerful. When you love yourself as *you are* and not as *you wish you were,* you are freeing yourself from the thoughts, opinions, and expectations of others. Worrying about what other people think or being critical of yourself is a quick and easy way to drain all your energy.

Exercise will always be a way I show love for myself. When I'm plugged into what my body is doing—pushing myself and leaning into the discomfort—I find it easier to process my emotions and manage my stress. I've felt unbridled joy when the instructor at a dance class encouraged us to "Let it go and dance our hearts out" during a Florence + the Machine song. The huge release I felt in that moment was an act of self-love. At a boxing class, when the instructor was yelling at us to "be a champion!" I let it all out at that bag and ended up sobbing. Pushing myself that hard showed self-love because giving my all made me feel so alive. Gardening does it for me too. Kneeling in the dirt, pulling out weeds so that my flowers and vegetables can thrive, is physically relaxing and reminds me that I have the ability to grow healthy food myself.

A big part of my self-love routine involves carving out time "to recover." Navigating a busy life takes energy. Exercise, whether it's walking, strength training, Pilates, or running, also takes physical and mental energy. To continue operating on a high level, it's important to take time for rest and recovery. Since I work out in my off hours as well as for work, I'm exercising twice a day (sometimes more!) five days out of the week, so proper recovery is essential. When we go hard, we need to compensate by also going easy. My recovery process includes everything from stretching and foam rolling to just spending an afternoon on the couch. I also love myself by booking a service that will help my mind and body recover from everything I ask it to do. Once a month I'll book a massage, see my acupuncturist, or go to physical therapy or Rolfing (fascia work). How we choose to express self-love is personal, but it should be something that makes you light up inside and soothes your body. Have a few go-to activities that invigorate you and make your soul smile. Self-love should be *a constant* in your life too. This isn't something you only pull out after a rough day to make you feel better. Imagine self-love as ongoing kindnesses that keep you energized and feeling good.

TREAT YOURSELF

Treating yourself is the act of doing something *just for you* because you matter and deserve special things. These are small pleasures we give ourselves as a reward or for no reason at all. Sometimes a treat might be as simple as a long bubble bath or buying a new book by your favorite author. A treat could be buying flowers at the grocery store and taking the time to arrange them in a vase on the kitchen island. Those flowers can serve as a reminder that you matter. When you look at those flowers you are *thinking of you* in that moment, even if no one else is. Sometimes a treat for me is making a cup of tea and sitting in my indoor jungle with Kimchi and Rhody. My interior jungle is like a sanctuary to me—the combination of the plants, my chair, my cats, and the view of the outside soothes me. Taking a few minutes to just be there feels special.

But my all-time favorite treats actually have nothing to do with calm and quiet. Dave and I love going to concerts and to hear live music, and this is an activity we've come to prioritize. We've gone to see the Red Hot Chili Peppers, ODESZA, *and* Khruangbin recently. Listening and dancing to music with Dave and my friends creates memories we will talk about for years. Every time we go to a concert, I leave buzzing with energy and thinking, *That was the best! Who will we see next?* I'm already looking forward to the next treat, and just thinking about what it might be gives me a boost. Treats are those special little things that stand out and make life pop. They are important reminders that there are always things to look forward to and good times to be had.

DATE YOURSELF

I started dating myself, and I have to be honest, at first it wasn't easy. Taking myself out wasn't exactly scary, but it was definitely awkward. We are so busy all the time, so scheduled and constantly connected, that being alone in a restaurant came as a bit of a shock. When I started taking myself out for dinner, I had thoughts about things I had never considered . . . *What do I do with my hands? Do I just stare at the wall? Will people think I'm a freak if I sit here quietly and just do nothing?* Resisting the lure of the phone was hard; it's such an easy out! But I wanted to be present, to enjoy the gift that is being able to go out for dinner and eat such wonderful things. I wanted to appreciate every single smell and subtle flavor, I wanted these evenings alone to be a gift to myself. Now, every Monday night I have a standing date with myself (and a big bowl of noodles). I've roamed the city eating up soba noodles, dan dan noodles, miso ramen, brothless ramen, wonton noodle soup, dumpling soup, tofu salads, pickled vegetables . . . ALL of the wonderful, beautiful food. While the food is the highlight, it's not the sole purpose of these outings. This is doing something for me and taking the time to fully appreciate and savor something I love.

The Japanese restaurant I'm taking myself to tonight is on a quiet side street in an otherwise ultra-busy Midtown Manhattan. I cross over the busy avenue onto the street that's graced with brownstones and quiet little restaurants. There is a short set of stairs leading down from the street, and when I enter the restaurant I step into a bundle of activity. Waiters scurry around carrying big steaming bowls of deliciousness. The restaurant is full of couples and groups of friends sharing conversation and noodles. I tell the hostess I'd like a table for one. She leads me to a table in the corner. The red decor gives the place a cozy feeling—like I've stumbled into a secret den for noodle lovers. She smiles and hands me a menu. "Just you?" I nod. "Yes, just me." She grabs the second set of cutlery off the table and scurries off to her next task.

I dive into the menu as I would a new book. I read about how they prepare the pork broth in some sort of special pot for hours and hours. I learn that "round blade noodles fineness #26" are a preferred noodle to use here, because it fits in so well with the pork broth and the chashu—or slow-roasted pork belly. In my head, I am drooling. I have no shame when it comes to noodles. While I am a ride-or-die noodle fan, the rest of the menu holds my attention too. Edamame, shishito peppers, three kinds of hirata buns—chicken, pork, and veggie—and sake cocktails. I decide on the classic ramen (fineness #26 for the win) and start with the ohitashi— seasonal chilled veggies in dashi dressing. After I order there's always a bit of awkwardness for me. It is almost laughable how difficult it is to know what to do with yourself when you're alone. At first, I always revert back to checking my phone, even though I tell myself to just be. Just sit! I use the time to scroll through my emails, answering some and making notes about things I'll need to take care of later. I put my phone down on the table and have to force myself not to pick it up again. Smartphones are such a default—such an easy way to distract yourself from aloneness.

The ohitashi arrives—it's practically a work of art. Carrots, daikon, broccoli, peppers, and cauliflower all cut into perfectly proportionate shapes. There is nothing basic about this. They are as colorful as a kaleidoscope, presented in a mason jar, which I gently pour onto my plate. They are tender and flavorful—the dashi dressing adding a crazy amount of flavor, but not overpowering the simplicity. They are so pretty, I am almost sad I'm alone just because it would be nice to share the loveliest vegetables I have ever seen with Dave. I tell myself I'll have to bring him the next time we are in the city. The ramen arrives next, the flavor of the broth practically detectable from the steam rising off of it. The bowl in front of me might as well be a bowl of pure joy. Give me a bowl of noodle soup and I'm basically a kid on Christmas morning. A bowl of noodles has the power to relax me, excite me, nourish me, and make me feel like the world is just the most wonderful place and it is *just good to be alive*. I dig in with my chopsticks, going straight for the noodles. They are a perfect texture, a hint of a bite but not al dente . . . and definitely not too soft. The noodles carry the flavor of the broth along with them, rich and meaty with the ideal level of saltiness. The chashu practically melts in my mouth like some kind of magical not quite liquid gold. I taste it all, feel it all, and am appreciative for the hands in the kitchen that crafted these noodles, created the stock, roasted the pork so well. I eat slowly and deliberately, finally shedding the self-consciousness of being alone, because now I am grateful that there is nothing else for me to do but marvel at all of the beauty inside of this bowl.

Time alone for just you and something you love is an incredible gift to give yourself (even if it's a hard gift to accept at first). Have you allowed yourself time to truly be alone? Just you, no smartphone, nothing but you and your five senses. It's so incredibly easy to be distracted, to not enjoy experiences fully because life is constantly flying at us. We don't have time to smell the roses, much less the bone broth that's simmered for sixteen long hours. But carving out time each week, even if it's just a super quick activity at first—to savor a perfect cappuccino, to walk in the woods, to order a single glass of pinot noir at a wine bar, to see a movie, to browse in a bookstore without being rushed . . . this is some of the greatest love you can show yourself.

The term "self-love" is thrown around a lot, but how many of us really put it into practice in a consistent way? What would it be like to put these concepts into action by purposefully loving, treating, and dating yourself? We spend so much time caring for others and navigating the day-to-day demands of life that we don't often take a moment to give ourselves props for a job well done. Self-love means knowing your value, and something starts to shift inside when we acknowledge that value. We revel in our self-worth, understand our strengths, and become aware of how much we're capable of. When you love yourself the energy you put out into the world sparkles and shines. Loving yourself is like having your own stash of secret treasure. You walk through life knowing you're worthy of the wonderful things that come your way. While I had loved myself and treated myself consistently for a long time, it never occurred to me to take myself out on dates. But something started to shift in me after I added noodle dates to my self-care routine. I shed the anxiety about being alone; I didn't care if I was essentially staring at a wall. The simple kindness of taking myself out overshadowed all that, and all that was left for me to do was eat and enjoy. That's the real power of self-love, it puts you in the right frame of mind to enjoy what's right in front of you. Love yourself, treat yourself, date yourself . . . and get ready to relish all the goodness and joy *you bring* into your own life.

SIXTEEN

Progress Is Forever

The ninety-mile bike ride along the coast of Japan was one of the longest rides I had ever done, and it was definitely the most beautiful. Dave and I rode past acres of rice fields that were about to be harvested. The bright green and neon-yellow grasses in the rice fields were blowing in the wind, almost like they were cheering us on. We rode along miles of rocky ocean coastline, with steep cliffs plunging down to the crashing waves. Everywhere we looked there were mountains in the distance. Even the rest stops on this ride were special. There were none of the typical protein bars and energy drinks you usually find during events like this. Instead, we were given rice balls, mochi, and noodles . . . some of my very favorite foods. When we finished the ride we checked into our hotel and discovered it had a hot spring. It was the perfect place for Dave and me to rest our legs and recover. As I let the hot water both calm and recharge my body, the magnificence of this trip was fresh in my mind. "Dave, this has been so amazing. I'm sad it's over." Dave and I had always wanted to go to Japan, and this opportunity to collaborate with a travel company on this trip was a dream come true. Dave looked at me. "Emma, I'm sad to leave too. But we've seen such amazing things and there is just so much more for us to see out there in the world. Who knows where we'll go next?" As I finally pulled myself out of that hot spring (you should have seen my crazy sunburn), I realized that while this chapter of my life was ending, my story had a very long way to go.

I returned from Japan and threw myself back into my life—going back to work at Peloton, writing a blog post summarizing our trip, cleaning up my garden as the summer ended, and, most notably, putting the final touches on this book. As I sat at my desk, overlooking the garden Dave and I created together, I realized that we are constantly faced with endings. Trips, jobs, workouts, dinners with friends, dance parties, concerts, and gardens all come to an end. There is that moment when all of the excitement and anticipation we've had about something is over . . . the event has happened. It's done. More than anything, writing this book and visiting Japan have shown me that these special moments don't just end—they position us for the next chapter.

Dave and I were thrilled when the opportunity to travel to Japan came up, but we were a little scared too. We are adventurous travelers, but it's not easy traveling to a country where not only can you not speak the language, but you also can't read a single street sign. Dave and I went out for ramen one night. Our hotel had recommended a place and we were keen to try it. We ventured out into Tokyo, carefully following the directions to the best of our ability. As we stood on a corner, trying to find the right street, Dave pointed down a narrow alleyway. He was trying to compare the characters on our phone to what was on the sign, "Emma, I think it might be down here?" We carefully walked down the alley, wondering if we were completely off course. Toward the end of the alley, we encountered what appeared to be a tiny restaurant. "Could this be it?" We compared the sign to what was on my phone, and it seemed to match. We walked into a warm, clean, and spare place, where we were welcomed kindly by the proprietors, who'd been eagerly awaiting us. I ordered ramen with all of the toppings . . . an egg, mushrooms, bamboo shoots, seaweed, scallions. The steaming bowls of ramen with truffle miso broth tasted otherworldly. We had traveled to the other side of the world to discover that there is no limit to how supremely delicious noodles can be. Since Japanese cuisine is probably my favorite to eat, I was excited about the long traditional kaiseki dinners we would have. Each little dish set before us was more beautiful than the last. There were many tiny bowls of flavorful dishes; there was a sizzling pot filled with homemade silken tofu. There was a grilled fish, pickled vegetables, and expertly prepared monger eel. Monger eel has thousands of tiny bones throughout, and only a well-trained chef knows the proper way to cut the eel in diagonal angles to break all of the bones enough so you can comfortably eat it. Finally, the meal was topped off the way we begin a Japanese meal in the States . . . with miso soup and rice. The food was beautifully crafted and prepared with care, like everything we encountered in Japan, and I wondered, *Will I ever be able to prepare food like this myself? It's so gorgeous! So much attention to detail!*

The trip only got better. We visited a Buddhist temple where we had the opportunity to meditate with monks. I loved the bells and the gongs. Sitting and breathing next to monks who have dedicated their lives to the practice of meditation was a huge privilege. We visited a knife factory in Sanjo-Niigata, an area famous for their exquisite work, and we were able to make our own. The craftsmen who taught us have been refining their craft for over forty years. There was so much skill and honor in what they do. We also got to visit an Iaido dojo. We put on traditional garments and spent an hour learning different katas and working with an unsharpened sword before we got to hold the real deal. When a samurai sword was placed into my hands, I immediately felt its weight. I needed two hands to hold it. There was more to its weight than just heft; it came with the gravity of long traditions and great craftsmanship. As I swung at the rolled-up wet tatami mat (they have about the same density as a human leg) I was in awe of what I was holding. As I whacked off the top of the mat, I wondered about the sword in my hands. *Who made it? What was his story? . . . What were the stories of his people?* I loved everything about Japan, from the gracious people and the food (even the 7-Elevens have rice balls!) to the beautiful parks and the cleanliness of the subway. I was moved by the way the Japanese people take care of their country and their culture as a way of showing respect for each other.

Back home I sat at my desk putting the finishing touches on this book, and I started to feel a twinge of anxiety. How do I end a book about my life when it's just begun? How do I know when it's really finished? What if I didn't always choose the best words? What if I left out a crucial story? As I began to stress about all this, I let my mind wander back to Japan. It was hard to believe that just a few days ago I had been sleeping in a traditional ryokan and doing my best to sample every interesting beverage offered in the great vending machines of that country (there was even hot creamed-corn soup!). I started to realize that while I would "finish" my book, my story will continue to evolve and grow. Like the Buddhist monks and samurai sword makers in Japan, my book (and my life) was an example of *progress not perfection* in action. Those monks can't ever achieve a perfect state of meditation; they wake up every day and engage in the process; they meditate to progress. Those craftsmen don't spend forty years working on one perfect knife—they focus, learn, and get better over time. *Getting better never has to end.* My entire life has been and will continue to be about progress. Perfection isn't just an unattainable ideal, it suggests that there's a final ending. Perfection suggests there is nothing more to do, and I want to do more. Progress means there is always more to do, there's always something new to see, learn, or eat. While I poured my heart and soul into this book, it's not the end. I have more living to do, more stories to tell, and more noodles to enjoy.

I left Japan knowing so much more about a new culture and even hungrier for new adventure. I write the final words of this book appreciative of how much I've learned about myself and knowing there is so much more I'd like to experience. Progress is what gets us all to the next place, and progress also leaves us room to take wrong turns and make mistakes. If Dave and I had misread the sign of the ramen restaurant, we might have ended up in a different restaurant eating the most fabulous sushi of our lives. Or worst-case scenario? We would have gotten totally lost and just scooped up a couple of rice balls at the 7-Eleven. It's a story we probably would have laughed about for years.

I've been writing this book for more than a year, reflecting on my roots, my culture, my family and friends, my relationship, my home and garden, my passion for fitness and love for food. I could go on forever, but at some point, you have to stop. I know this book will never be perfect, but that's because nothing is. Perfection is an ending, and I'm not interested in an end. I'm interested in what happens after you turn the last page. I want to hear the story about how you feel after you crush a goal and set a new one. I'd love to hear about your next trip to a faraway place! But I also want to know what you learned from it, how it impacted you, and where you're going next. Progress is a lifelong pursuit, and I'm committed to enjoying every beautiful, messy moment of it all. I might be about to finish this story, but there is so much more to explore and so much more to do. I don't know what my next chapter will be, but I'm open to whatever it brings. As we all turn this last page, we have the power to jump into another story. When you push perfection away and embrace progress with your whole heart, you're opening yourself up to endless possibilities. Explore those possibilities and enjoy them, but most of all relish the knowledge that there are countless stories to be lived. You just have to get out there and live them.

ACKNOWLEDGMENTS

Thank you, reader, for trusting me with your time and opening your heart to this book. To Hilary Teeman, thank you for believing in me and for that initial phone call many summers ago that sparked this entire journey. And to the rest of the Penguin Random House team, Caroline Weishuhn, Kara Welsh, Jennifer Hershey, Kim Hovey, Lindsey Kennedy, Abdi Omer, Jennifer Garza, Debbie Aroff, Jordan Hill Forney, Ada Yonenaka, Belina Huey, Julie Ehlers, and Janice Race, I appreciate you!

Thank you, Paula Vitale. You are talented, funny, and honest, and that is exactly what I needed in order to tell my stories. This would not have been possible without you. I value your ability to ask the right questions and listen without judgment, and your overall vision that made this book come alive. I also appreciate your similar love of noodles. Thank you!

Dave. Thank you for your patience, love, and support, forever and always. And to Dave's family, Sue, Shannon, and Libby, for being there for me and for us.

My Vineyard ladies, Mariah, Emily, Tonya, Kelly, Fiona, and Elizabeth, you have my heart. More than anyone else, you have all seen me change and grow, and I honor the bond that we have created over many decades of friendship. To John, Jei, and Nate Thayer for being a part of the village that raised me. And to Dianne and Tom Durawa, my godparents, who have shown nothing but support through all of the successes and difficult times.

To my family, Mark, Teresa, Alan, and Jenn. I love you and I'm so lucky to be related to you. Thank you for allowing me to share our stories. And to my niblings Luca, Alani, and Nico, the world is your oyster and I love being your auntie. Speaking of aunties, I must thank all of mine and my uncles for supporting me and always cheering me on. To my Po Po, none of this would be possible without you. You are resilient and wise, and I thank you for being you.

Thank you to my UTA team, Brandi Bowles, Byrd Leavell, Lauren Nogy, Ali Berman, Nicole Vincent, Max Stubblefield, John Seitzer, and Shelby Schenkman, for making so many of my dreams come true! And to Thomas Li for your enthusiasm and time spent on the newsletter/site in between saving lives. Thank you, Emily Beal, for supporting me and Live

Learn Lovewell in all of the incredible ways that you do. You help to make it all happen!

To my Peloton colleagues and teammates, in front of the camera and behind the scenes, thank you for showing me what hard work and greatness look like. John Foley, thank you for your creativity and innovation, and for taking the chance on me from the Kickstarter campaign to Instructor. Thank you, Robin Arzon (*New York Times* bestselling author), for taking my phone call and heading up the team as fiercely as you do. The way you lead by example has been an inspiration to me for many years. Jen Cotter, I appreciate your leadership and encouraging me to always shine brightly. Thank you, Tunde Oyeneyin (author of *Speak*), who I got to watch thrive in the launch of her book and who never missed a moment to be a resource and a friend to me throughout this journey. To all of the Peloton members who have sweated with me and rocked out with me class after class, I appreciate your continued support and celebrate you in all that we have accomplished together.

Kimchi and Rhody, my fur children, you make life so much more hilarious and cuddly, and I love you for that.

LIVE
LEARN
LOVE
WELL

Emma Lovewell

Random
House
Book Club

Because
Stories Are
Better Shared ™

A BOOK CLUB GUIDE

QUESTIONS AND TOPICS FOR DISCUSSION

1. Has perfectionism affected your life? Do you ever feel pressure to "get yourself together"? If so, how do you generally go about accomplishing that? What did you learn about the difference between progress and perfection? How will you live intentionally in progress rather than perfection?

2. Discuss Emma's attitude toward her mixed-race ethnicity and how it informed and shaped her into the woman she is today. How did being mixed race impact her experience growing up?

3. We all have a bad habit that we rely on to get us through tough times. What's one in your life that you'd like to eliminate to better your health and overall wellness?

4. Emma states that when grieving it is "so tempting to

numb ourselves during difficult times, with alcohol, food, or even flat-out denial." How do you deal with grief in your own life?

5. Emma shares many personal stories and anecdotes in this book. Did learning about her struggles and triumphs impact your view of how fearlessness can be achieved? How so?

6. Emma discusses being comfortable with your true self, which isn't always easy. Do you feel confident in who you are and where you are in life? If so, when do you feel this the most?

7. What does unconditional self-love look like for you on a daily basis?

8. Did this book spark any additional ideas for change in your life?

9. Emma became a lip-sync champion at a young age with her rendition of Mariah Carey's "Dreamlover." What song would you have chosen to lip-sync to in a competition as a child? As an adult?

10. Emma talks about how saying "yes" can create abundance and new opportunities in your life. If there was no fear, what would you say "yes" to?

11. Peloton fans: Which of Emma's classes is your favorite? Why?

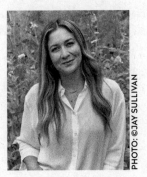

PHOTO: ©JAY SULLIVAN

EMMA LOVEWELL is the founder of Live Learn Lovewell, a Peloton instructor, an Under Armour athlete, and an all-around health and wellness expert who is dedicated to teaching others how to feel good in their bodies and live their best lives.

Livelearnlovewell.com
Instagram: @emmalovewell
X: @emmalovewell

ABOUT THE TYPE

This book was set in Sabon, a typeface designed by the well-known German typographer Jan Tschichold (1902–74). Sabon's design is based upon the original letterforms of sixteenth-century French type designer Claude Garamond and was created specifically to be used for three sources: foundry type for hand composition, Linotype, and Monotype. Tschichold named his typeface for the famous Frankfurt typefounder Jacques Sabon (c. 1520–80).